WINNING AT WEIGHT LOSS

Achieve your slimming goals, enjoy food & feel great again

Books by the Speakmans

Conquering Anxiety

THE
Speakmans

WINNING AT WEIGHT LOSS

Achieve your slimming goals, enjoy food & feel great again

First published in Great Britain in 2019 by Orion Spring
an imprint of The Orion Publishing Group Ltd
Carmelite House, 50 Victoria Embankment
London EC4Y 0DZ

An Hachette UK Company

1 3 5 7 9 10 8 6 4 2

Every effort has been made to ensure that the information in the
book is accurate. The information in this book may not be applicable
in each individual case so it is advised that professional medical
advice is obtained for specific health matters and before changing
any medication or dosage. Neither the publisher nor authors accept
any legal responsibility for any personal injury or other damage or
loss arising from the use of the information in this book. In addition,
if you are concerned about your diet or exercise regime and wish
to change them, you should consult a health practitioner first.

A CIP catalogue record for this book is available from the British Library.

ISBN (Trade paperback) 978 1 8418 8323 6
ISBN (eBook) 978 1 8418 8324 3

Printed and bound in Great Britain by Clays Ltd, Elcograf, S.p.A

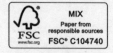

www.orionbooks.co.uk

ORION
SPRING

Important Information Before Reading this Book

This book is not a substitute for physical activity, or medical, nutritional or psychological intervention, nor is the content intended to replace therapy, dietary advice, exercise regimes or medical help and advice.

We are confident that this book will help to positively alter your perspective and attitude in relation to eating, weight and weight loss, and make a significant positive difference to your relationship with healthy eating and exercise; however, there are no guarantees.

If you feel that you may have medical issues as a consequence of obesity, an eating disorder or have any other health concerns, we would recommend speaking to your GP for advice.

It is a good idea to seek the advice of a health professional before starting on any weight-loss programme, as they can also advise you about useful local services, such as weight-loss groups and facilities, where you may be referred to a health team for sessions under the supervision of a qualified fitness trainer and registered dietician.

If you have a weight issue that you feel may be due to a health concern, your GP may recommend tests or specific treatment.

If you're unsure of your health status, have multiple health problems or are pregnant, speak with your doctor before starting a new exercise or eating programme.

We would always strongly encourage you to speak with your doctor or health professional about how you are feeling, and also to enquire about therapy, should you feel that you need emotional help and support.

Contents

Introduction

We have helped thousands of people to attain their weight-loss goals, to feel great and to transform their lives, and are excited to guide and support you through every page of this book to help you do the same. This is an area that interests us greatly, because we have seen for ourselves the positive repercussions that come from repositioning and conditioning negative schemas, which can imprison people within their own minds and bodies. Although we will explain this in more depth later in the book, in brief a schema is a thought process or a learning from experiences in our life, that then goes on to be a reference for future behaviour. We have followed the transformational journeys of those who have benefited from our personally developed 'Schema Conditioning Psychotherapy'® and now we would like to share that with you.

We understand the frustration you may feel when overeating, the internal conflict and the desperation to regain control. We understand because we have been where you are, both personally and professionally. The realisation hit home to us when someone mentioned how lucky we were to be 'naturally' slim. In fact, we have lived and breathed our approach every day for over two decades. We, too, have been on the journey of self-analysis that we are about to guide you through. The results for us and our clients have been life-changing, and we would now like you to add your own success story to ours.

You were great, you are great, and we want to help you look great and feel great, too.

Everything you do starts with a thought. Whether you overeat occasionally or often, the fact is that you have NEVER eaten anything by accident, and this is our area of expertise.

If you do overeat or have weight issues or an unhealthy relationship with food, the question that needs to be answered is: why and when did this start? You see, you were not born overweight. Something happened; something changed and caused you to see food differently. This, we believe, is the missing component in achieving your slimming goals. It is also the component that is consistently overlooked and the area that excites us, as it is so powerful in reprogramming your eating schemas.

In this book we would like to share with you the approach we have successfully used with our clients who have battled weight issues and the internal conflict of not wanting to overeat, while at the same time feeling powerless to resist.

So why is it that when you know the downfalls of overeating, when you know that it's detrimental to your health and you would feel happier looking healthier, you still continue to eat unhealthy foods to the point of nausea or discomfort, promising yourself that from Monday you will go on a diet or start an exercise regime, knowing full well that Monday often never comes, or certainly never lasts?

We are going to help you find the answer by guiding you through a simple process of self-analysis, in order to better understand your behaviours and to locate those negative behavioural schemas that trap you in a perpetual loop of dieting and overeating. Our aim is also to help you challenge your negative schemas and reposition the memories from your past that affect your future.

The UK National Health Service states that obesity reduces life expectancy by an average of three to ten years and contributes to at least one in every 13 deaths in Europe.[1] We do not want you to become one of these statistics, and therefore we are excited to share with you our schema conditioning therapy and weight-loss formula, including some effective tools and simple techniques to help you enjoy food and feel great.

We want to offer you answers to your behavioural patterns associated with eating. We want to help you see food in a healthier and more positive way. We want you to feel in control and to take control. We want to help you unravel why you overeat, and then to help you sever your obsessions with food to enable you to establish a healthier, happier life.

We are here for you. We believe in you, and know you deserve to be happy. Together we will embark on your journey towards health using our tried-and-tested approach to winning at weight loss.

> 'Take care of your body. It's the only place you have to live.'
>
> **Jim Rohn**

1

Our Therapy

Nik and Eva Speakman saved my relationship . . . with FOOD!

Well, I suppose it started when I was a baby. I was always regarded in my baby photos as a podgy, cute wee baby. I imagine that back then it was a term of endearment. However, in my childhood and then my teens, I was far from podgy, though I still had the label. I was now a skinny wee thing. During that period the food was provided for you, either by your family or your school meals (with no famous chefs giving advice) – certainly very few children in my day cooked, except for some ghastly concoction that you made in home economics and took home to the family, who devoured it lovingly. Healthy eating was a salad of lettuce, a hard-boiled egg and a tomato with a slice of processed cold meat . . . and if you were lucky, some salad cream.

So when I became an adult and could make choices, I did, but they weren't the right ones. As I grew from a teenager to a young adult with a job that included business lunches, any thoughts of healthy eating flew out of the window, and yes, the weight just piled on and on.

Oh, don't get me wrong – I saw it happening, and I tried to do something about it. Diet drinks. Diet foods. Diet clubs. Diet books. Diet magazines. Gym memberships. I tried them all, but with no long-term success. I lost weight, got a badge . . . dropped a dress size, then put it ALL (plus more) back on again. I was in a downward spiral, and it was not a happy time until . . . I met Nik and Eva.

I went to a seminar that they held called Winning at Weight Loss. This was the start of my new relationship with food, which has continued for over four years. This seminar was THE best event I have ever attended. Nothing that requires effort is ever easy, but until you understand your relationship with health and food, you won't understand how you can change.

Nik and Eva give you the information, the tools and techniques to take you on your own personal journey to happiness. I know that if I had not attended that seminar my life would still be the same: I would be overweight, with health issues, and not happy with my appearance and lifestyle as a result.

They approach this topic in a way that lets you decide what you need to change and how you can go about changing it. Food and health are no longer a worry, and you really have nothing to lose . . . well, I did – I had three stone to lose, and you know what? I haven't put it back on, it's stayed off. I perhaps am not considered 'skinny', but I feel at 64 that I am okay.

I can now enjoy wearing make-up, buying clothes, eating. I love food, but it's the right kind of food, as Nik and Eva showed me, and I don't miss the unhealthy things that were ruining my life. I still have the odd treat – of course I do – but why ruin my life after it was saved by Nik and Eva? They did not just change my relationship with food; they changed my relationship with LIFE, for which I will be forever grateful.

Thank you, Nik and Eva . . .

Wendy, with love x

Everything Starts with a Thought

We know that everything we do starts with a thought, and therefore this book is about understanding, managing and addressing the thoughts – or schemas – you have created during your life that cause you to overeat and sabotage your weight-loss success. It's also thoughts that create your perception of yourself, food and eating.

Our hope for you in reading this book is that you will get to experience our therapy. We would therefore like to start our journey together by explaining the basis of our approach in a personalised way that you can identify with. Once you understand this, you can relax and know that we will share information and suggestions with you, to help you see food from a different perspective. When you accept this new perspective, the way you look at food should change and, in turn, your relationship with overeating should change, too.

Finding the Cause

With that in mind, to help explain our approach to weight loss, we would like to share a metaphor with you. Imagine that you have a frequent itch on the back of your neck. The area itches, and so you scratch it, which gives you temporary relief, only for the itch to resume again a little later, which makes you feel frustrated.

You show the site of irritation on the back of your neck to your family and friends, and they assure you there's nothing there to see, yet the area continues to itch, and as much as you really don't want to, you cannot help but scratch. The urge is too strong, and so you give in.

You feel too embarrassed to seek medical advice about your itch, as you do not want to trouble your doctor with something that seems relatively trivial, so you attempt to resolve the issue yourself. You try various things to address the itch, such as applying creams, changing your laundry powder, trying different clothing fabrics and changing your fragrance and body lotions, but to no avail. Each effort fails, regardless of what you try, and the itch persists, leaving you feeling disappointed and upset.

Eventually you go to see your doctor, who assures you that there is nothing on your skin, therefore it's likely just an irritation, and so you leave the doctor's surgery with advice to try all the things you have already tried. You feel frustrated and sad. The itch dominates your thoughts and weighs you down. You enjoy scratching the itch in the moment, but then immediately feel exasperated and annoyed that it persists. You try to ignore it, but the itch wins and you cannot stop yourself scratching, and so the cycle resumes.

Then, one day, you bump into us and you tell us about your irritating itch. You tell us you wish you didn't have it, but that the moment you feel it, you can't help but scratch the area furiously.

And so we say to you that all we want to know is when did it start, and where is the location of the itch? You tell us you recall it starting at school when you began to wear a school blouse with a collar, and the origin of the itch is on your neck. We then ask if you have ever considered cutting the labels out of the back of your clothing? You feel surprised that no one has suggested something so simple before, but realise that the origin of the itch each time is exactly where your clothes label is and that it started at a time when a clothing label would have been in close contact with your skin for the first time, and for prolonged periods.

This new perspective gives you hope, as it makes sense, and as soon as you cut the labels out of your clothing, the itch stops. In that moment, your need to scratch immediately disappears, as the cause of the itching has been addressed.

Although this is a simple metaphor, we have found that, just as scratching is the symptom and the clothing label the cause in this example, the need to overeat is also a symptom, behind which lies a cause. Just as you don't want to scratch, equally you do not wish to overeat, but you get a strong urge that you feel you cannot control. And once you've scratched or eaten and the moment of need has been satisfied, there usually follows a feeling of guilt, disappointment or frustration.

Our therapy is based on helping you locate the cause of your overeating, and positively changing the schema behind it – just like discovering it was your clothes labels that caused you to scratch – so as to help your weight-loss journey.

The Solution

Knowing the cause of your overeating, however, is not enough. Once you have identified the event and the belief (behavioural schema) you created that now prevents you from losing weight, you have to take action to address them.

Throughout this book, we will help you by offering suggestions and sharing real-life examples and case studies that you may identify with, so that you can apply our formula to yourself and your own personal circumstances.

Within our metaphor, we helped you locate the cause of your itch, and you then had to go home and physically remove all the labels from your clothing. Altering the schema or schemas that prevent you from losing weight is similar. There are actions you will have to take, which we hope to make as simple and clear as possible.

The good news is that, once an offending schema has been positively conditioned with the overwhelming evidence we provide, the need to overeat should dissipate – just like that itch. The process is just as straightforward as our metaphor would suggest. The itch analogy is a great example of how our therapy works and how you can change without needing multiple meetings with us to keep reminding you to cut the labels out of your clothes. We are often told our work and approach are simple, and this is a great compliment.

> **'The definition of genius is taking the complex and making it simple.'**
>
> **Albert Einstein**

Once your schema has changed, it alters how you feel. Every one of us has a number of negative schemas, and we want to help you discover yours – in particular those that prevent you from achieving your slimming goals.

Our Questionnaire

So, welcome to your first session with us. We all have 'itchy labels' that cause us to adopt negative behaviours that need to be addressed, so let's find out more about you to help you discover what life events may have created the negative schemas that today stop you from losing weight. At this moment you may not even realise or believe that a particular event in your life – from your childhood, your teens or some point in adulthood – could contribute to your inability to lose weight, but as you read through our book, you will learn how past events can impact your future.

You have probably never studied or dissected your life to locate the origins of your overeating, your anxieties, your fears, your issues, your low self-esteem, your need for protection, your need for love or your need to be overweight. You have probably never considered whether you could have a behavioural reference or schema that causes you to overeat, such as: 'being big keeps me safe'; 'being big stops me from standing out'; 'being big helps me to belong'; 'being big prevents me from having to face emotional pain' or 'I must eat now as food could be scarce in the future'. These are just a few examples of schemas we have come across over the years as we have been helping people with their weight-loss issues. Schemas are often created as a consequence of a life experience, which then goes on to cause people to struggle with weight loss.

We would now like to help you look for clues as to what the origin of your schema might be, as well as consider positive elements of your life, which can be overlooked but are equally important in your quest to win at weight loss.

It's important to note here that reading this book alone will not resolve your issues and stop you overeating. You must participate in the exercises we share, just as we would expect you to do in a session with us. So please take a pen and a notebook to use as your 'winning journal', and write down your answers to the following questions:

* **Briefly describe your typical day. What do you do?**

* **Who are the people you surround yourself with? People can hugely impact how you feel, so it is very important to consider this.**

* **Who do you spend most of your time with? List family members, work colleagues and friends you see the most, and note below each name:**

* **Does this person have issues around overeating themselves or are they constantly dieting?**

* How does this person make you feel about your issues with food? Do they support or sabotage your weight-loss efforts?

* Looking at the friends and family you have listed above, note how you would expect them to react or behave towards you if you were to reach a healthy weight and maintained it effortlessly? Would they still be your friend? Would they feel proud? Would they feel insecure?

* What events, people or experiences have contributed to making you the way you are today? Please be specific. List the positive. List the negative. (As you read through this book, these are potentially the schemas you will need to address and challenge with contrary evidence.)

* When you think of each negative experience above, give a score out of ten for your feeling about that person or event, ten being the worst feeling and zero being no bad feeling at all. If you have a highlighter, highlight this question, as when you have finished reading this book and have worked on each event, you can score each one again to show what has changed and what still needs to be worked on.

* What would you say are your biggest personal:
    1. successes?
    2. failures?

* When you think of each failure above, score your negative feeling about it out of ten. Highlight this question, so that when you have finished the book, you can note how each failure has resulted in a positive learning experience.

* What is your specific reason for reading this book? Noting and rereading this every time you pick up the

book will help you to look for a solution to this specific problem. It will also keep you motivated to win at weight loss.

* When did this issue start? Knowing this will give you a clue as to when in your life something may have occurred to create your need to overeat.

* Were your parents, siblings, close family members overweight, or did you grow up observing someone who had issues around food? If so, who?

* In childhood, were you rewarded with food?

* In childhood, were you told to clear your plate? Were there consequences if you did not?

* Were food and treats plentiful or insufficient when you were a child?

* As a child, did you have siblings or family members who would eat all the treats if you didn't get to them first?

* Have you ever been bullied in your life? Consider schoolmates, parents, siblings, partners, spouses, work colleagues and teachers.

* Please write beneath anyone you have listed above the primary hurtful things they would say, or how they made you feel, particularly in relation to your size, height, weight, image or abilities.

* Did you grow up being discouraged to be yourself? Or discouraged to be in a relationship with the person of your choice? If so, who discouraged you and how did that make you feel?

* What dreams and ambitions did you have when you were younger?

* What dreams and ambitions do you have now? This will help you to reflect on the things from childhood you may still like to work towards as an adult.

* List the values and qualities you appreciate about yourself.

* Score your life out of ten. Highlight this question and please reflect on this again when you have read the book, considering what other actions you can take to make this score a nine or ten.

* If you could attempt any one thing and you knew that you couldn't fail, what would it be?

* Finish the sentences below, writing the first thing that comes to mind:

'Life is a ....,'

'People are ....,'

'I am ....,'

'I need ....,'

'I wish ....,'

'If only ....,'

* What is your most frequent recurring thought? This will give you an idea of what occupies your mind – it may also be creating your need to eat, so needs to be challenged.

* List everything in your life that you appreciate. Please highlight this question and, from today, read your list each morning to help you to start your day in a more positive way. Add more things as they spring to mind.

* List your top-ten personal successes (e.g. passing your driving test, earning a degree, getting married, getting a job, organising a party, making someone laugh, an act of kindness). Read this list each morning, along with the list of all the things you appreciate in your life.

* What comedians/actors make you laugh? You can't always control external events, but you can make time for laughter, and watching clips of these people will help you feel happier, therefore reducing the need to overeat for comfort or creating feel-good hormones.

Your Timeline

To help you identify potential triggers from your past that today contribute to preventing your successful weight loss, writing a timeline of significant events in your life can be an effective tool. It can help establish the causes of your schemas and forms an essential evidential component in our therapy.

As you read this book, we will encourage you to focus on the negative events in your timeline and to positively change your perspective on the contributory schemas. We will direct you to these negative events and to points in the questionnaire you have just completed at the end of each chapter, and then help you to address each of them one at a time.

It is equally important to be aware of all the positive things that have happened in your life, which should include your achievements, times you have laughed uncontrollably, been somewhere exciting, fallen in love, had an amazing date, been to a fantastic concert, and other memorable events. You should read over the positive events on your timeline regularly to remind you of the great things you have done, seen and experienced.

To try to reduce the detrimental effects of each negative memory or past event, it is important to find an element of positivity within it, to help you feel better about it. This may be acknowledging that you have learned something new from it, or that it made you stronger, more empathetic, kinder, or better able to help somebody else as a result.

Also, if the event is something that has been and gone, consider that it is therefore now over and you are no longer a victim of it; you survived it and you became a victor.

Alternatively, you can change your emotional attachment to a negative event by accepting that it was not personal to you. For example, if you have experienced an abusive relationship or bullying, consider that this was not instigated by you, nor was it personal to you – the abusive partner or bully will have been abusive to others in the past and will continue to be abusive to others in the future. The abuse was not because of you, it was because the abuser had an issue. As bullying is a common cause of weight issues, we will cover this in more detail later in the book.

If, after reading this book and considering its suggestions, you are still struggling to change a negative event by viewing it from a more positive perspective, try speaking to a therapist or a friend that you trust. Explain to them that a painful memory is affecting you, and ask if they could offer any suggestions that would help you to see the event in a more positive light, so that you can sever that negative emotional tie and leave the event in the past.

Clearing the Past

We want to help you work through all your negative life events slowly and systematically. Even those events you may not feel are relevant to hindering your weight loss may have a bearing, as food is often unconsciously used as a form of self-medication.

As you process each negative life event one at a time, move on to the next one only once you are starting to feel better, so that you can work through your painful memories methodically until they have no residual negative effect – or at least a lesser negative effect – on you today.

Carrying the past around with you is an unnecessary weight on your shoulders that has a detrimental impact on your life. Therefore, even if you find it difficult to lessen your negative emotions, you can start by making the decision to remind yourself that what you endured should not have happened, that you didn't deserve it to happen and that it is now over. At the very least, a timeline like this is a great tool to take with you if you are undergoing therapy, as you can direct your therapist to all the areas in your past that you would like to work on.

Furthermore, going back to our earlier metaphor of the clothing label being the cause of your incessant and uncontrollable itch, if that were a real scenario and we suggested that the likely culprit of your itch was the clothes label on your neck, even before cutting the labels out of your clothes you would have immediately felt hopeful and encouraged. Therefore, as you look at your questionnaire and timeline, please feel hopeful and encouraged that you are now discovering the fundamental causes of your negative eating behaviours and starting to address them.

Now, using the template overleaf please complete a timeline of your life events. We send out timelines along with

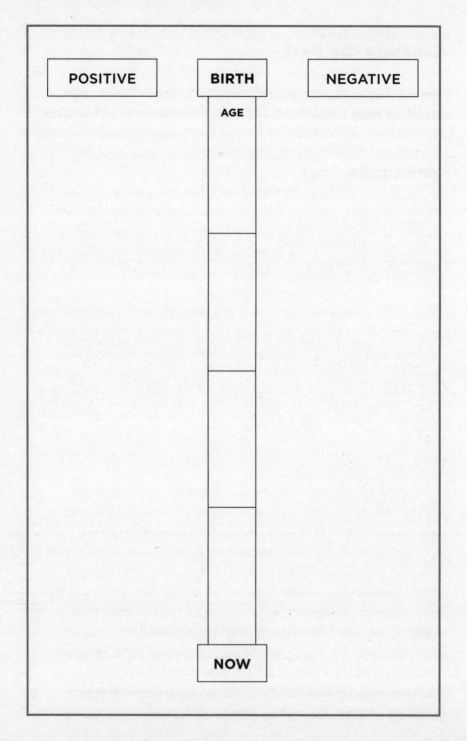

our therapy questionnaires to all our clients, and often we receive more than one page back – in fact, one lady sent us 17 timeline pages, as she had so many life events to deal with. Bearing that in mind, do not worry about how many pages you fill, as long as it allows you to find the answers you need.

Healing the Past

Researchers found that middle-age and older women who experienced more stress from major life events were more likely to develop obesity than women who did not report any stressful events.

Live Science[2]

Once you have written your timeline, consider each negative event and whether it still affects you or causes you any discomfort or anxiety. Score the negative event out of ten (zero means it has no negative effect and ten means you feel an extreme negative reaction).

If you have scored a six or above for anything in the negative life event column, this could be contributing to your weight issues, because you may have created negative behavioural schemas for which food is your go-to comfort. These are the events that need to be challenged by positively altering your perception of them, in order to condition the schema that you created at the time.

See it for what it was and not how it felt.

If you can see an event for what it really was and not how it felt at the time, this will allow you to become emotionally distanced from it. You can then become a third-party observer of that life event, as opposed to allowing the memory to play in your subconscious and affect your present. You will notice, for example, that when your friends have a problem, although you may be upset for them, you are personally detached from the issue, which allows you to maintain emotional objectivity, to soothe them and forget what happened. This is where we want you to be when you think about any negative memories you have, so to help you begin, we would like you to go through each negative event in your timeline and ask yourself the following questions:

* **Was it personal? For example, was someone mean just to you or were they unkind to everyone? If so, realise that the event was not specifically about you. Perhaps the person who made you feel bad had low self-esteem or had a difficult upbringing, so they knew no different. Perhaps they felt unhappy with their image, so tried to drag you down to give themselves a feeling of superiority or power.**

* **Was what happened just an unfortunate accident?**

* **Could it have been a misunderstanding? If so, how might you have misread the situation?**

* **What did you learn? Did the event make you stronger, wiser, more compassionate or able to help others?**

* **What good came from that? Did the event make you more charitable, more understanding of others?**

* **What actually happened? Describe what happened – factually and without emotion.**

None of us is immune from bad things happening, and we often get trapped in a past event without realising that we had no control over it, forgetting that, despite this, we survived it.

Traumatic life events can often feel personal and make us feel lonely and weak, but please know that you are not alone. We have all had life challenges – some worse than others – but take solace in the fact that, despite everything, you got through all your issues. You survived your worst ever day, and therefore you can get over any other issue, too, and go on to inspire others and make those who love you happy and proud.

You may not be able to forget the event, but you can certainly change your perception of it, cut the emotional ties and therefore achieve your slimming goals, so that you can enjoy food and feel great again as a result. Furthermore, doing so should encourage more positive thoughts to surface. Past negative life events overshadow many of the happy memories we hold. Therefore, once negative schemas have been lifted, good memories are able to shine through.

You deserve to be happy, healthy, in control and achieving your weight-loss goals. So, a very well done for taking the necessary action to start working on your thoughts and feelings, so as to improve your relationship with food.

2

What Are Overeating Disorders?

An eating disorder is when you have an unhealthy attitude to food, which can take over your life and make you ill. It can involve eating too much or too little, or becoming obsessed with your weight and body shape.

National Health Service (NHS) UK[3]

In this chapter we would like to share with you a little more information about overeating disorders, which may sound familiar or relevant to you. We will also share some examples of their origins to help you start to unravel the unwanted eating behaviours, food 'addictions' and eating patterns that inhibit your slimming goals.

Surprisingly, at the time of writing, obesity is not included in the range of classified 'eating disorders' on the NHS website. However, in our opinion, whether it is overeating, bingeing or undereating, if you are unable to maintain a balanced way of eating, and obsess about eating, not eating and your weight – all of which can be incredibly distressing and frustrating for you, your family and loved ones – then this is essentially an eating disorder.

Eating disorders are not only about the way a person perceives food and behaves around it, but also about their underlying thoughts and feelings. We have helped many people who have struggled with an overeating disorder, and have seen first-hand the distress, frustration and sadness that comes with any difficulty in achieving weight-loss goals.

For many, an overeating disorder may be a way of coping with painful or negative thoughts – a form of self-medicating, self-sabotaging or self-harming, or a way of feeling in control. However, again, in our experience, every eating disorder (except perhaps 'rumination disorder', which we reference on page 36) is a symptom, behind which lies a cause. Negative or self-destructive behaviours are often a reaction to a difficult life event, and together we want to help you find the missing piece in your weight-loss journey.

A Barrier to Happiness

When you are battling with weight loss, you are often also struggling with the additional weight of anxiety that no one else can see. This mental and emotional burden can sometimes feel heavier than the extra physical weight you carry, as you try to avoid photographs, social events, beach holidays and even eating in front of others whom you feel judge you and watch over you with disapproval. This emotional pain can lead you to sabotage your own weight-loss goals, adding even more to your overeating disorder.

> *To change the behaviour resulting from a behavioural schema, the behavioural schema has to be changed.*

Bulimia

Famous faces who have openly spoken about their battle with bulimia include Paula Abdul, Russell Brand and Princess

Diana.[4] People who have bulimia go through periods where they binge-eat a large quantity of food in a very short space of time, and in an effort to rid themselves of what they have consumed, they will then make themselves vomit. After a binge, the individual may feel guilty, fat, anxious and sad. Bulimia often goes hand in hand with low self-esteem.

There are numerous health implications associated with bulimia, which can include irregular periods or no menstrual cycle at all, a sore throat from vomiting, tooth decay as a consequence of stomach acids affecting tooth enamel, heart disease and a host of bowel and colon issues if using laxatives.

I have been suffering with my body image, low self-esteem . . . You have given me the tools I need. I feel wonderful and grateful that I was able to speak with you at your workshop. I feel fantastic.

Mikki S

CASE STUDY
Isabella: Bulimia

Isabella had come to the UK as a student from Eastern Europe and was living with an English family: Adrian, Terri and their children. Terri was becoming increasingly concerned about Isabella's eating habits.

Over the months, Isabella became part of the family, babysitting when the host family were out for the evening and forging a great friendship with the children. However, the family were unsure how to approach Isabella with their concerns, not wishing to upset her, push her away or admit that they had done a little detective work in her room while she was out. This left Terri feeling disloyal, despite having only good intentions.

Terri became aware that Isabella was in possession of a large volume of laxatives. She also saw discarded shopping receipts in the waste bin, confirming purchases of laxatives and large quantities of junk food. Terri explained to us that she had become so conscious of Isabella's issue that she had developed a heightened awareness of everything Isabella did around food.

Not wanting to be accused of being a snoop or to break the trusting and solid relationship she had formed with Isabella, Terri was unsure what to do. She even considered making contact with Isabella's mother in desperation. However, Terri then decided to book onto one of our workshops and to obtain a ticket for Isabella, in what she could pass off as a 'treat', in the hope that, if there were an issue, perhaps it would encourage Isabella to acknowledge it and ask for help.

During our workshop, we spoke about confidence and self-esteem, and how many people struggle with both – often as a consequence of having been bullied or made to feel inadequate at some time in their life. We went on to touch on the possible consequences of these negative life events, which included overeating disorders such as bulimia and binge-eating. Unbeknown to us, our words were touching a nerve for Isabella, and when we asked for a volunteer to demonstrate our confidence-building technique (shared later in the book), she bravely raised her hand.

As she joined us on the stage, Isabella told us how she felt she had lacked love as a child growing up, primarily because she had lots of siblings and both her parents spent many hours at work. As a consequence, she had quickly immersed herself in a relationship with a young man at college, giving him every ounce of her attention. She explained that, over time, he had become aggressive and possessive, and made her feel she was fat, stupid and useless.

Your opinion of yourself is based upon how other people have made you feel.

As we asked Isabella to look in the mirror on our stage and describe what she saw, she used degrading, disrespectful words about herself. We later asked how many of the words she was using had been based on the words of her ex-boyfriend or the way he had made her feel. Isabella cried as she confirmed that it was 'most of them'.

We helped Isabella to see herself through the eyes of love (we share the process in Chapter 8, page 148) and to realise and appreciate her true worth. We asked her to consider any possible motive her ex may have had to destroy her self-esteem. She shared that all his previous girlfriends had cheated on him, and that perhaps he was punishing her for their mistakes. We pointed out that if his girlfriends cheated on him, this would probably have knocked his confidence, and thus it was more likely that by making Isabella feel bad about herself, she would feel worthless and lucky to have him as a boyfriend, and would therefore be less likely to stray.

This resonated with Isabella. She accepted that she was a beautiful and kind person, both inside and out, and that in hindsight the fact that her ex had tried to make her feel bad about herself was likely – as we had intimated – to prevent her from straying. Isabella agreed that his fear of losing her proved that he must have felt she was too good for him.

Isabella walked off stage to an enormous round of applause, with her shoulders back and her head held high. At the end of the workshop, Terri made her way over to speak with us. She explained to us why she had brought Isabella to the workshop, and told us of her suspicions that Isabella may have an eating disorder, such as bulimia. She also told us that after she had come off stage, Isabella had hugged Terri and thanked her, and at the next break, she had admitted to Terri that she had been (in her own words) 'self-harming' by eating huge amounts of high-calorie foods and then using laxatives and making herself vomit. She saw herself as fat and ugly, and feeling bad about herself would make her want to eat junk food, after which she would feel disgusted with herself.

Terri promised that she would update us on Isabella's progress, which we received some months later. Terri wrote: 'After the workshop, Isabella had a spring in her step. Your workshop allowed us to have an open and honest conversation about Isabella's issues around food and eating, which in turn allowed me to be able to offer her my help and support.'

If the cause is the foundation, the symptom is the structure. If the foundation is removed, the structure falls down.

Avoidant/restrictive food intake disorder (ARFID)

Avoidant/restrictive food intake disorder (ARFID) is a pattern of eating that involves the restriction of certain foods, though not as a result of wishing to lose or gain weight. ARFID is often a repulsion, fear or inability to eat certain foods due to a negative or unpleasant association with them. The smell, texture or look makes the sufferer feel completely unable to even try the food.

When we have been faced with someone who has ARFID, it has most often been described to us as 'a phobia' of eating certain foods, with the majority of people having a diet orientated around only high-calorie foods, such as chips, yoghurt, chicken nuggets and toast, which in turn resulted in poor health and an inability to lose weight.

This food avoidance causes great angst for many, as they find themselves unable to socialise or participate in activities that may include the foods that they feel unable to face. ARFID can be detrimental to one's health, as it can prevent the sufferer from eating important nutrients that the human body needs.

For some, ARFID can actually lead to weight loss; for others it can lead to extreme weight gain and obesity, such as a lady we met who could not eat anything that contained or had come into contact with fruit or vegetables, including sauces and gravy. Her diet consisted of chocolate, fried chicken, chips, bread and cheese.

Everyone we have personally met suffering with ARFID has developed this eating disorder as a consequence of traumatic events, including choking or vomiting, leading them to develop a fear of the same thing happening again, and thus avoiding those foods altogether.

We discuss food phobias and anxieties in more depth in Chapter 11. As food restriction can lead to extreme health issues, it is important to seek treatment as soon as possible.

CASE STUDY
Bradley: Avoidant/Restrictive Food Intake Disorder

Bradley had experienced issues with trying new foods from childhood. Now, in adulthood, his diet, social life, health and unhealthy weight gain were worrying him.

We asked Bradley whether he had any idea why this issue had started, and he told us that his mum had noticed a change when he started nursery school. Bradley did recall memories of being taken to nursery by his mum at lunchtime for his afternoon sessions. He would be placed at a round table with lots of unfamiliar faces, and Bradley recalled crying for his mum while having food pushed in front of him.

Bradley wondered whether this was the reason why now, as an adult, he could only eat childlike foods such as chicken nuggets, chips, crisps, beans, spaghetti hoops, bread, burgers and toast. Living off these high-calorie foods was taking its toll and Bradley was desperate for our help.

We presented Bradley with a tray of foods, including fruits, vegetables and chicken, and asked him to explain his feelings. He shared that the thought of the foods made him feel uncomfortable, anxious and distressed.

We explained to Bradley that, in view of what he had told us, it appeared that at nursery, he had created an inaccurate negative schema linking his heightened feelings of distress and abandonment at that time to the foods that had been placed in front of him.

We highlighted to Bradley that he appeared to be using this inaccurate childhood schema, and was in essence consulting his child self on how to react to new foods as an adult. His response was, quite literally, childlike.

To condition Bradley's schema, we asked him to consider why he was choosing to blame new foods for his mother having to leave him at nursery. We asked how food could be responsible. He confirmed it was not.

It was also vital that we added a positive element to his nursery experience, and therefore we asked him to consider why his mum had taken him to nursery. How might it have assisted his mum? How might it have assisted his development? Bradley went on to say that nursery had allowed his mum to work and to care for him, and he had also met his best friend at nursery, who he is still friends with to this day.

After addressing all the benefits of nursery and of healthy foods, and allowing Bradley to laugh at the fact that he had blamed food unfairly, making it a scapegoat for his feelings of abandonment, we then carried out our Bungee Technique (shared later in the book, see page 167) to positively alter Bradley's coding of new foods. We were then ready to test whether Bradley's schema had been conditioned.

Again, we presented Bradley with a tray of fruit, vegetables and chicken breast. This time, although apprehensive, Bradley was willing to try some of the new foods before him. He was only taking very small bites, and needed encouragement to chew and swallow them, but slowly he started to build his confidence. We explained to Bradley that he would need to continue building on his confidence in this way, but we were thrilled that he had been willing to try new foods.

This was a new experience for Bradley and we advised him to take his time and to experiment with new foods slowly to create new adult behavioural schemas orientated around food. He emailed three months later to tell us that he was becoming more confident with food and was now enjoying new, healthier choices, which he was certain would lead to weight loss.

> *Learning to walk, you fell many times, but never once did you give up on learning to walk.*

Other specified feeding or eating disorder (OSFED)

Any eating disorder which does not exactly fit the criteria of others falls into the category of OSFED, or 'other specified feeding or eating disorder'. Symptoms can vary, and can include elements of other eating disorders, such as temporary or occasional bingeing, overeating, undereating or food avoidance.

Some conditions that fall into the category of OSFED include:

NIGHT-EATING SYNDROME

Night-eating syndrome (NES) is very common. This is where someone eats a lot of food after their evening meal or wakes up during the night specifically to eat. Many people with NES feel like they have no control over it, and often feel ashamed or guilty the next morning, with good intentions for the new day ahead, which they rarely manage to see through. People with NES often consume the majority of their daily calorie intake after their evening meal. Common causes of NES include not eating regularly throughout the day, overly restricted daytime food intake, lack of good-quality sleep, loneliness, boredom, tiredness, stress or unresolved emotional issues, which we look to address in this book.

RUMINATION DISORDER

A person with rumination disorder regularly regurgitates their food. In essence, this condition is the backward flow or resurfacing of recently eaten food from the stomach to the mouth. The food is then rechewed and swallowed or spat out. The cause of this condition is not fully understood, although it is likely to be biological, possibly due to a build-up of abdominal pressure.

PICA

People with pica regularly eat things that are not food and have no nutritional value, such as chalk, metal, ice, sponge, ash, paint and even hair. Pica is a compulsive eating disorder, and is believed to be more common in children, affecting 10 to 30 per cent of young children between the ages of one and six. Apparently, pica can also occur in children and adults with autism. On rare occasions, pregnant women crave strange non-food items, such as dirt,[5] chalk or ice, which is believed to be related to an iron and or zinc deficiency.

We have worked with people affected by pica on a few occasions. The cases we have encountered have primarily involved hair eating and sponge eating, which has been triggered by a specific event. Fortunately, in these cases, we were able to help the sufferers control their compulsion by helping to address the traumas that led to it, such as grief and heartbreak, as well as supplying them with lots of evidence as to why their behaviour could be harmful to them.

PURGING DISORDER

People with purging disorder try to influence their weight or body shape by using laxatives, diuretics, excessive exercise or fasting, but they do not binge-eat. It is believed that purging mainly affects women, with up to 70 per cent of sufferers also having a mood disorder, and up to 43 per cent having an anxiety disorder.[6]

People who purge have similar feelings to those who suffer from bulimia or binge-eating disorder, and often feel guilt and shame. They therefore do not always admit they have a problem or ask for help, which of course they should.

BINGE-EATING DISORDER

According to Beat, the UK's leading eating disorder charity, a 2015 study conducted by Hay et al. found that binge-eating accounted for 22 per cent of eating disorders.[7] Binge-eating is probably a condition that many people who struggle with weight loss can relate to; plenty of us have 'binge-eaten' at some time, as it is often the consequence of unresolved emotional issues.

If you experience binge-eating disorder, you might use food to cheer yourself up, to fill a void, to distract yourself, for comfort or even as company when feeling lonely. In our experience, binge-eating disorder often goes hand in hand with people who are stressed, anxious, have low self-esteem or who have faced numerous life challenges.

Binge-eaters feel out of control with their eating, and therefore often feel ashamed and embarrassed. There can also be numerous negative health consequences with binge-eating disorder, particularly weight gain, diabetes and high blood pressure.

CASE STUDY
Lily: Binge-eater

Lily, a fashion designer, told us that although she did not consider herself to be ridiculously overweight, she was incredibly frustrated, as she knew she could look better, feel better, weigh less and be healthier. However, her issue was that when she ate or drank anything that she would consider a treat, such as a cake, biscuits, crisps or sweets, she could never just have one or two – she would always consume to excess.

If she decided to have some chocolate, she could never just buy one bar; she would have to buy three or four, and would have to eat all of them all at once. She felt this bingeing was her biggest hindrance in achieving her weight-loss goals.

We explained to Lily that we are all a product of our environment, our individual life learnings and our experiences. We therefore believed that her bingeing behaviour was a symptom, which must have an underlying cause. We shared with Lily some possible causes based upon those of people we had helped in the past. These examples included:

1 A feeling of famine learned from childhood, if you grew up in poverty or in a house with a lot of other children where you had to often go without. This then elevates the status of sweet or 'treat' foods.
2 A home with siblings where competition existed for 'treats', encouraging a 'greed' behaviour.
3 You felt the weakest, odd one out, or you were an only child and so ate for comfort.
4 You were the eldest sibling, and you had younger brothers and sisters at home. When you came home from school, there were hardly any treats left. This again could instigate a behaviour of bingeing so as not to go without.

Immediately Lily identified with this. She said, 'I can't believe it, as that is exactly what it is; I have a younger brother and sister and there is quite a big age gap between me and my younger siblings.' She went on to say, 'I do know that I would often come home from school, Mum would have been shopping with them during the day, buying nice things for us, but there would be hardly anything left.' Lily told us that if she was ever around when her mum bought anything, she would eat it really quickly – as much as she could – as she knew that if she didn't, her siblings would eat it.

Lily was flabbergasted. She said that this really felt correct, that this was exactly what had created her bingeing behaviour, but that she had never realised it before.

We knew that this information alone would give her a different perspective on her eating habits, as she could now understand and rationalise that they were originating from something in her past. However, a quicker and easier solution was to positively condition Lily's schema, so to do this we put some questions to her:

'Do you still live with your brother and sister?'

Lily said she didn't. She had a flat in London, while the rest of her family lived in the Midlands.

We then asked: 'Is there anyone in your flat who would eat your food while you are at work?' Again, Lily confirmed that she lived on her own, therefore the answer was no.

We asked: 'When you were a little girl, who bought the treats?' Lily replied that it was her mum.

We then asked: 'Who buys the treats now and who is in control of who can eat them?' Lily laughed and said, 'Oh, yeah, that would be me.' We asked Lily what that might suggest to her. She confirmed that if she wanted to have more treats, she was completely in control of that, and that she did not need to rush to eat everything, as no one else was there to eat them.

Lily said that she felt very silly but very happy with this revelation. Later that evening, we received an email from Lily to say that she was delighted because she had popped into a store at the train station to get a snack, and it was the first time ever that she had bought just one small chocolate bar, rather than feeling compelled to buy lots more, even after eating it.

We bumped into Lily at a function a few years later. She looked fantastic and was so happy to see us. She gave us the hugest hug and told us that her bingeing days had left her when she had left us.

3

The Speakmans' Schema Conditioning Psychotherapy

Feeling utterly repulsed by chocolate and crisps now thanks to the Speakmans and the treatment they shared at their workshop. I haven't eaten chocolate. I've been offered it and actually said no! Wow is all I can say. Wow!
Michelle

In this chapter, we will share the method that we use when working with clients who are suffering with issues that lead them to self-medicate with food. We want to help you address the origins of your overeating. We hope to help you remove any barriers you may be hiding behind, to dilute your insecurities, to boost your confidence and self-esteem and to positively change your perspective on painful past memories that may be contributing to your need to overeat. We want you to realise your potential and embrace your future, free from the burdens of the past.

> *Life is for living, and to enjoy it, you need to be healthy.*

We believe that, deep inside, everyone knows the person they would love to be, the life they would love to live, and, more importantly, that they deserve it. Yet happiness and emotional peace can seem unattainable, with numerous invisible barriers, negative thoughts and beliefs, uncontrollable compulsions, fears and anxieties preventing us from living that life.

How Does Our Therapy Work?

Many people comment, having observed our therapy and work – whether in person, at our workshops, on television or via the films on our website and our YouTube channel – that the solutions to the issues people present to us often appear simple. In fact, we hear frequently that 'surely it can't be that easy'. The truth is that, usually, it is quite straightforward to resolve an issue and alter a negative behavioural schema, once you know how. We hope that by reading through the many successful case studies within this book, you will find personal resonance that will enable you to address your own negative behavioural schemas and apply our formula to your issues.

Often, because we are at the centre of our own problems, anxieties, fears and insecurities, we are unable to see things impartially. We are so tangled up in our issues that we do not have an objective or advantageous view point. For example, if you are driving on a road and become stuck in traffic, you are unable to see any side roads or alternative routes in advance that will get you out of that traffic jam. Whereas if you were distanced from the road, seeing it from above, for example, you would have a better view and would see exactly where the roadblocks are, what to avoid and the quickest way to get to your destination.

Sharing the case studies of the people we have helped is like giving you that distanced, elevated view, which will allow you to see other people's issues from a third-party perspective. We find this process very effective in our clinic, which is why we want to share it with you, too. You will see similarities between the issues and events in other people's lives and your own, and having no emotional ties to the case studies will allow you to absorb the formula we have used with others and apply it to yourself.

Since [being] with you guys I have so changed my thinking. I'm even now thinking of stepping out of my comfort zone. I worried what people would think, but you amazing couple have made me think so differently and positively. I now believe I can do things regardless of what others think. Love you both.

Sharon

As you will see from the case studies we share, we usually manage to help people within just one therapy session. The reason why we have such a fast and positive impact is because our clients complete a very detailed questionnaire prior to meeting us. From this, we are able to understand the potential life traumas and events that may have caused our client to turn to food in adulthood, and we can then prepare a personalised therapy session for them.

Conditioning Your Negative Schemas

We want to make addressing and changing your negative schemas simple. This amazing process of overcoming past issues that lead you to overeat or have an unhealthy relationship with food should be as straightforward as possible, so that you can get on with the important job of living your life, making yourself happier, feeling more fulfilled and allowing your life to flow more easily. However, there is work involved on your part. Once you have our formulas, suggestions and information, we pass the baton to you, asking you to use them to challenge your own life and your own schemas (beliefs/behavioural references). After all, we update our smartphones regularly, making sure they are running on the latest software and functioning at their best. How amazing would it be if everyone had that same determination to upgrade their own thought processes, beliefs and behaviours to create a healthier life?

So, take a few moments now to consider how your relationship with food is stopping you from achieving the things you want and from being the person you want and deserve to be – a healthier, fitter person who is in full control of their life.

You will undoubtedly harbour behaviours from older operating systems and ideas you had when you were younger, but as with your phone, it's time to upgrade your operating systems – your schemas – to give yourself the best life possible – one in which you are not shadowed by guilt, embarrassment, frustration or shame.

The Speakman Way

'To enjoy good health, to bring true happiness to one's family, to bring peace to all, one must first discipline and control one's own mind. If a man can control his mind, he can find the way to Enlightenment, and all wisdom and virtue will naturally come to him.'

Buddha

A schema allows us to organise and interpret information. It is a learned or copied pattern that becomes an automatic reference for how we think, act and ultimately behave. In our therapy, we help to locate negative schemas that are a result of past negative life events. These may have evoked emotions such as fear, envy, embarrassment, grief or shame. We then help our clients to mentally reposition the memory of the event in question, thereby upgrading its negative emotions to positive ones.

The therapy that we have developed over the last two decades is called 'schema conditioning psychotherapy' (not to be confused with 'schema therapy', a different type of therapy that we do not practise).

Schemas direct our behaviour

In 1952, psychologist Jean Piaget defined a schema as 'a cohesive, repeatable action sequence possessing component actions that are tightly interconnected and governed by a core meaning'.[8] In simple terms, schemas are the basic building blocks of intelligent behaviour and a way of organising knowledge. You could also think of schemas as files containing vast amounts of information, which are stored within the filing cabinet of your memory. Each file tells us exactly how to react when we receive incoming stimuli. Schemas are 'learned references' that allow us to be proficient in everything we do – from brushing our teeth to driving our car; from how we communicate with ourselves and others to how we react to a spider.

For example, we all have schemas for what to expect from having a meal in a restaurant. The schema will be a pattern that includes looking at the menu, choosing your food, ordering the food, eating it and paying the bill. Whenever you are in a restaurant, you will run this schema, and just like a computer program, it will run in the same way every time.

The blank canvas of new life

We are born a blank canvas – **tabula rasa.**

Every healthy, typical brain has the same lack of knowledge at birth. As we grow up, we learn from our parents, extended family, friends and peer groups and from our own individual experiences of our surroundings. The way we personally process the world dictates how we see ourselves and our environment, and how we behave and react to any event or situation that we are faced with.

We are all born with a small number of innate schemas. These are the cognitive structures underlying our reflexes. For example, babies have a sucking reflex that is triggered by something touching their lips, and a grasping reflex that is stimulated when something touches their hand. Most schemas, however, are learned – as a result of copying the behaviour of our parents or people we're in close contact with, or through our own interpretation of personal life experiences.

Developing schema conditioning psychotherapy

Having trained in various fields of therapy over 20 years, we identified that we had great skill in helping people change their mindset and behaviours just by talking with them and encouraging them to look at situations from a different perspective.

We believe that people possess inner wisdom, and via our talking therapy we are able to tap into this, to help them find a new understanding of why they think and behave the way they do, thereby changing their negative schemas. This is the foundation of our therapy and we passionately want to share with you the secret to finding what is often the missing component to healthy weight loss. The good news is that the power to control your eating, weight and health is within you.

> *There is a misconception that we use some kind of magic, hypnotherapy or confusion methods, but our therapy is no more than a straight-talking conversation, leading to a cognitive restructure of negative schemas.*

A simple change in perspective

Overeating is driven by your negative schemas – but all schemas can be changed. Here's a simple example of how.

Imagine your favourite restaurant, where you go most weekends, as the food is consistently good and you are never disappointed. There then comes an occasion when you order your favourite meal and it's not up to the usual standard, and you leave feeling disappointed and unfulfilled. You assume that this is just the chef having an off-day, only to return the following week and find that once again the food is substandard, and you leave still feeling hungry. You try one last time, only to learn that the old chef has left, so you no longer return to this restaurant, as your schema about that restaurant has changed.

You now have a negative schema about the restaurant, and you would require a lot of overwhelming positive evidence to return to it.

Changing your mind

Another example of how schemas can instantly be changed or 'conditioned' is if you have always liked a particular food, such as tuna fish, but then one day you are very sick after eating it, and each time you vomit all you can taste is partially digested tuna. This new negative association provides you with an alternative perspective on tuna, and your schema changes immediately. As a result, your behaviours and feelings towards eating tuna also change. Essentially this is how our therapy works: we help to change your perspective forever by providing new, overwhelming evidence. However, unlike with the tuna analogy, in which the association changed from positive to negative, our skill is in applying overwhelming positive evidence to a negative schema, which provides an alternative perspective very quickly. We then effectively and precisely deliver that evidence to the person we are helping. These are the five steps we use to condition negative, destructive or unhelpful schemas. Follow them to alter your unhelpful schemas, too.

1   Using your timeline, find the original event that has caused your negative behaviour around eating. Remember that you may have more than one event that now leads you to struggle with overeating, so concentrate on tackling and positively conditioning just one event at a time.

2   Once you have located the event in your timeline, question how you interpreted that event at the time. How old were you, and how did you perceive the event at that age? Consider how your perception then could have been flawed or inaccurate, now that you can see it from an adult's perspective.

3 Collate contrary evidence to positively condition your perception of the event and your resulting schema. If you find it difficult to challenge your current belief, ask a friend whom you consider wise and positive to give you an alternative perspective. We will give you many examples of this in the case studies within this book.

4 See the event for what it was and not how it felt. If you were a third party and this had not happened to you personally, how might you have seen it differently? What do you need to think and feel to sever your emotional tie to that event? Again, you will see examples of this throughout this book to help you.

5 Decide to be a victor, not a victim. If things from your past continue to affect you then you are still a victim of that person or event. Make a decision today that you will be the victor of your past: you survived it and you are prepared to alter your perspective to set yourself free.

Everything you do starts with a thought, even eating!

4

The Speakmans: Winning at Weight Loss

I'm blooming amazing. I'm feeling so free and at the moment I am just happy. I'm losing 1 or 2lb a week because I'm not doing the 'diet', I'm changing my lifestyle. It feels so much nicer than the pressure I'd normally put on myself.

Ashley

In this chapter we would like to share with you what we believe are the necessary components for achieving weight loss, including our philosophy and approach towards it.

A symptom

Over the years, we have helped many people change their perspective on eating, as well as their mental and physical health. This has led them to alter and improve their relationship with food, which has in turn encouraged weight loss.

However, we understand that to overeat to one's detriment, to be unhealthy, to be overweight and suffering the associated health issues, is not a conscious choice. In our experience, the battle of weight loss and the conflict of overeating to excess is a symptom, behind which we have always found a cause.

The principles of weight loss are straightforward: eat less

and move more. If you don't use up the energy food gives you, then your body will store it as fat. Therefore, if you eat more calories than you need to, your liver will convert carbohydrates, sugars, protein and fats into fat. This fat is then stored in fat cells until you need energy, when your body will use it, unless it has a quicker source, such as something you have just eaten.

The ubiquity of high-calorie temptations, the pressures of everyday life and a lack of sleep are all contributing to 64 per cent of adults in England being either overweight or obese.[9]

Seeing something new can be as easy as turning your head in a different direction.

Physical health

We've all heard phrases such as 'use it or lose it' and 'move more, eat less', but actually, for many, exercising is a struggle. For some, going to a gym is too intimidating or too pricey. For others, health issues prevent the possibility of any exercise. Lack of time or too many other responsibilities also feature as common excuses as to why people cannot exercise. However, as long as there is any trace of a negative association with exercise, there will also be a barrier. This will then lead you to look for excuses as to why you can't exercise, as opposed to focusing on reasons why you can.

Many of us have what feels like an automatic default, whereby we justify to ourselves why we cannot or should not exercise today. However, we must also consider that we are living a much more sedentary lifestyle these days, so our redundant fat stores are being added to – for some people, on a daily basis! We no longer walk to the local shops, carrying bags of shopping and fresh produce home each day. We can now drive to the supermarket, and if that sounds too strenuous, we can order food online and have it delivered right to our door. We no longer even need to walk into a restaurant or fast-food establishment, with drive-through facilities and home-delivery options available at the touch of a button. Is it any wonder, therefore, that as a nation we are gaining weight and our health is declining, with someone in the UK having a heart attack every seven minutes and a stroke every 12 minutes?[10]

Despite the fact that exercise releases feel-good neurotransmitters, so does eating delicious food, and given the choice, most will opt for the latter, as it requires less effort and can work alongside other pleasurable activities, such as relaxing on the sofa watching television or socialising with friends.

Analysis found that the average man in the UK spends a fifth of his lifetime sitting – equivalent to 78 days a year.

BBC/British Heart Foundation[11]

With worrisome statistics suggesting that 20 million Britons[12] and 82 million Americans[13] are inactive to the detriment of their health, we need to take action – now more than ever.

While exercising is a fast-track solution to increased health and weight loss, and most of us know it, for many, the prospect of physical activity still seems about as exciting as watching a radiator cool down. Later in the book, therefore, we will share with you some simple ideas and techniques to help you become more motivated to be physically active, in an effort to make this a strong part of your slimming process.

The prevalence of obesity in the UK has trebled since the 1980s . . . If trends continue as forecast, by 2050 only one in ten of the adult population will be a healthy weight.

The NSMC (National Social Marketing Centre)[14]

Environment

It is highly likely that you have not considered how your environment might affect your ability to achieve your weight-loss goals. But similarly, have you ever considered why you have the accent that you have? Why you like the foods that you do? Why you played the games you did when you were a child? Why you support your football team?

The answer is that you copied. You copied the accent of your parents and the people around you. You like and take comfort from many of the foods you were given as a child, and you played the games that were popular with the kids that you hung around with. Why would you support a different football team to your parents? Especially if your father or mother were really passionate about them and even referred to the team as 'we'.

You will no doubt remember your parents telling you not to hang around with certain children. If you are a parent now, you may not want your children to associate with certain groups because 'they are a bad influence'. Children copy, but because we tend to like people who are like ourselves, even in adulthood we can still be influenced. You may not think that other people affect your behaviours, but consider the fact that, when you are with people who like to gossip about others, it is difficult not to get involved. Equally, when you are with people who are giddy and laugh a lot, you are more likely to join in with the fun.

With that in mind, as an additional support during this process, you should always be aware of the people you associate with regularly. What are *their* eating habits like? Are they supportive or would they sabotage your weight-loss plans? No matter how well intentioned you are, no matter how motivated and focused, you should also be mindful of your environment and the people within it.

Sleep

Other environmental factors that can negatively impact your weight-loss success can include a lack of sleep. If you are sleep-deprived and tired, your body will naturally crave energy and search for a quick source, which is most easily accessed via carbohydrates.

Furthermore, when we are tired, higher levels of our 'hunger hormone', ghrelin, are released, while leptin – the hormone that tells us when we are full – is lowered. Therefore, irrespective of how focused and motivated you are to lose weight, a lack of sleep can cause you to overeat. If you struggle with insomnia, consider what the cause might be. Speak with your doctor and look through your timeline, too, as there could be clues there as to what is hindering your sleep. For example, if you grew up in a turbulent home, your sleep may have been disturbed as a child as you listened out for your parents arguing – you may never have addressed this or realised that, as an adult, you no longer need to be on high alert.

Biological factors

Hormones are enormously influential in how we feel, and as we have already mentioned, if you are producing too much ghrelin (the 'hunger hormone') and not enough leptin (the hormone that tells us we are full) then you will continue to battle with overeating to some degree. Although it may appear that hormone production is out of your control, there are numerous things you can try to counteract the effects.

A starting point should be speaking with your doctor, who can help you to balance your hormones if a biological or health-related cause exists. However, exercise, a healthy diet, herbal remedies, dietary supplements, acupuncture, meditation and reflexology can all help, too. We have both experienced hormonal imbalances in our lives that have affected our weight, due to thyroid issues and the menopause, and have used a combination of the aforementioned remedies to great effect. So be assured that a hormonal imbalance does not mean that you are destined to be horrendously overweight or that you cannot still successfully achieve your slimming goals.

Other factors

Life has ups and downs, and no one is immune to unexpected traumas or stress. At these times, we may turn to food as a short-term solution to feel a little better. It is important to realise that this is normal, and does not mean that you are a failure or that you cannot resume a healthy eating pattern.

> *We have all survived our worst day.*

Unrealistic expectations can sabotage your attitude to food and your attempts to lose weight. Accepting that it is okay to overindulge from time to time, or until the trauma or stress has dissipated or been resolved, is an important element in attaining in a healthier attitude to eating.

Everything you say, your body hears.

Alcohol can also significantly sabotage your healthy-eating and weight-loss intentions. When you drink alcohol the chemistry in your brain is altered and the neurotransmitters that process your thoughts, behaviours and emotions are detrimentally affected.

28.7 per cent of adults in England are obese and a further 35.6 per cent are overweight, making a total of 64.3 percent who are either overweight or obese.
Health Survey for England[15]

Dehydration can also contribute to struggles with weight loss, as even mild dehydration can make you feel hungry. The reason for this is that the same part of your brain is responsible for interpreting both hunger and thirst, and as a consequence of dealing with both, messages between thirst and hunger can often get mixed up. Known as the hypothalamus, this small area in the base of the brain performs many important functions, including the release of hormones and regulation of body temperature.

Mental health

No one consciously chooses to be overweight or unhealthy. According to the National Health Service, it is estimated that obesity and being overweight contributes to at least one in every 13 deaths in Europe.[16] This statistic is staggering, yet obesity figures and associated ill health and deaths are on the rise.

So why is it that so many of us do overeat and prevent ourselves from achieving our weight-loss goals? Many of us do not eat out of hunger, so why do we use food as a crutch when we're sad, mad, lonely, bored, disappointed, stressed – or experiencing any other emotion we can justify with a binge?

The answer to this question is different for everyone, but we believe it is the most vital component to successful, comfortable and permanent weight loss. Once you have answered this question for yourself, all your weight-loss failures, past and present, will be explained, and that inner voice that creates the conflict of wanting to lose weight while giving in to temptation will be silenced.

CASE STUDY
Gail: Low Self-esteem

Gail told us that she had grown up in a home where her father was absolutely in charge. No one crossed him, not even her mother. They would quake with fear if he were to become angry, or if she and her siblings made too much noise. Although he was a good provider, Gail would often observe her mum's subservience to her father, and would witness him being nasty, angry and controlling towards her. As a consequence of her conditioning, Gail assumed that this behaviour was normal and became far more tolerant of others being unkind or harsh towards her than she ought to have been. Her learning, or schema, had taught her that she should retreat and say nothing, and she quickly learned to sit and be quiet!

When Gail was 14, she met her first love, who went on to become her husband, and together they had three wonderful children. Although at the beginning Gail felt everything was perfect, once they were married and living together, she became aware that her husband was quite controlling. He did not allow her to wear clothes that he felt were inappropriate for her, and forbade her to go out and socialise with her friends.

Gail did her best to appease him, and would make excuses for his behaviour, but she was lonely. Her husband had a good social life, while she was left at home caring for their three young children. Once her children were in bed and her husband was out, Gail turned to food for comfort and company. She loved her husband, and was completely loyal, but after 11 years of marriage, she noticed he was spending less time at home. He began to pay more attention to his appearance, he joined a gym and his criticism of Gail increased. He also became more argumentative towards her. The knock-on effect was that Gail would eat more, and was gaining even more weight, for which her husband would berate and humiliate her. He called her vile names and made her feel completely useless. Gail said this was undoubtedly the hardest time in her life. Not only was her husband being unkind to her, but at that time her father was also terminally ill, so she could not even look to her mum for support. She felt incredibly lonely. The only friend Gail could talk to was another mother at the school gates, who she really appreciated; together, they would share stories of their woes.

One day, while her husband was showering, Gail spotted a text message coming through to her husband's phone. Her head began to spin and she fell to the ground, wanting to vomit. The message was from the mum she had been speaking to at the school gates, telling her husband how great their afternoon of passion had been earlier that day.

Gail felt like her world had completely fallen apart. The only two people she had thought she could trust had let her down. Gail felt like she had hit an all-time low. As soon as the affair came to light, her husband left Gail and she now spent each night at home, alone. All she had for comfort were cakes, sweets, popcorn and crisps.

Gail would eat until she felt sick, and then she would eat some more. Each morning, she would wake up feeling guilty about the amount of high-calorie foods she had consumed, and she would promise herself that the next day she would start afresh. She really tried hard to eat more healthily. She tried to follow diet plans and to exercise more, but she just felt like there was no point: she felt useless, worthless, pathetic, lost, cheated and humiliated, because her childhood sweetheart had not just let her down, he had shattered her whole life. She felt like a complete failure and believed that she was now too old to rescue her life from the mundane existence it had become.

Gail threw herself into looking after her children and helping her mother to care for her dying father, while she continued to gain weight. After six years of being single, Gail joined an online dating site. She had told herself it was just for fun, and she would never actually go on a date, but soon she started chatting with a man, who turned out to be amazing – so much so that, three years later, she married him.

Gail's new husband was a lovely man. He was kind and attentive and would pay her many compliments, which she would hear, yet never believe. As her children were growing up, Gail got a job and began to work full time as a carer. She loved the work, but her boss was quite unkind to her, belittling her in front of her colleagues. Gail did not want to make a complaint or bring it to anybody's attention, because the lady who was bullying her was in a managerial position and had been there a lot longer than she had. If there were any unrest within the workplace, the person they would get rid of would surely be Gail. She enjoyed her work looking after the elderly and did not want to jeopardise that in any way.

Gail's new husband loved her just the way she was, although Gail still consistently tried to lose weight and felt embarrassed by the way she looked. She said that she would never undress in front of her husband, as she was too ashamed of the way she looked, and if they went on holiday, she would always wrap up in a sarong. Despite her best efforts, she could just not maintain a healthy-eating plan, and would give an abundance of excuses as to why she was unable to exercise.

When we started to work with Gail, we wanted to understand how she felt about herself. We asked Gail to tell us what she saw when she looked in a full-length mirror. As expected, the words that Gail used to describe herself were very disrespectful. She used words such as fat cow, weak, pathetic, disgusting, disgraceful – all mean words that did not fit the kind-hearted soul in front of us. We did not believe that these words were her own; she was using the words of others to describe how other people had made her feel. It was heartbreaking.

When we asked Gail why she thought she was unable to maintain a healthy-eating plan and to follow a weight-loss diet, she actually said, 'I am just pathetic. I can't see anything through. I am weak-willed and I am an embarrassment' – feelings that made her get very angry at herself.

We did not think that this was the reason for Gail's inability to lose weight.

When we talked about her first marriage, we asked how that made her feel. She told us that it made her feel very embarrassed and ashamed, as everyone seemed to know about the affair except for her. She said that she had no doubt that people were laughing at her behind her back and probably laughing about how pathetic she was. Gail became upset and said that she had failed in her first marriage, failed to lose weight and that she was failing as a wife now, because even though she loved her husband, she couldn't even lose weight for him. During therapy, we are very attentive to the terminology people use to talk about themselves, as it gives us clues to the schemas that drive their behaviours. With this in mind, we both instantly believed that Gail's words offered the exact reason for her issue. It was clear to see that the word 'failed', which Gail used so often, was the cause.

We explained to Gail that the reason why she was failing to maintain a healthy relationship with food was because she believed she was a failure. We explained that, as long as she believed this, she would embark on a diet unconsciously expecting to fail, so that was exactly what would happen. Gail completely agreed that if she were honest, her efforts were half-hearted.

We spoke with Gail about her first marriage and asked about the vows she had made in church. When Gail repeated them, we asked her if she had failed her marriage vows. Gail confirmed that she hadn't – she had been loyal to her husband; it was he who had cheated on her and left.

We therefore asked her whether she had failed in her marriage. At first, she said she must have done, so we again asked her what she vowed she would do in her marriage. Again, she repeated her wedding vows. Again, we asked her if she had failed any of her wedding vows in any way. We pointed out that this was a yes or no answer only. Gail said no.

We then asked what she believed constituted a good husband and wife, and Gail repeated words such as loyal, kind, caring, loving, supportive and giving. Again, we asked her if she had fulfilled each of those roles as we repeated the words she had used back to her. She confirmed that she had.

We asked Gail again if she had failed in her marriage. This time, she said she saw where we were going with this, and replied no. It was refreshing to witness Gail as she, unprompted, started to tell us how she was a very loyal wife, and had her husband not had the affair, she would have stayed by his side forever. Again, we asked her to repeat whether she had failed as a wife and to repeat it in a full sentence. Gail said, 'I did not fail as a wife.' As she said this with conviction and certainty, we moved on to address her life now.

We asked Gail whether her husband gave her compliments. She told us her new husband gave her compliments all the time. We asked Gail whether her husband was a good man. Gail confirmed he was one of the nicest human beings she had ever met. We asked whether her husband was a liar, whereby she looked a little offended on his behalf, and told us, 'Of course not.' We asked Gail, 'If your husband isn't a liar, why do you call him a liar every time he gives you a compliment?' Gail replied by saying she didn't. We pointed out that, as she had told us that her husband gave her compliments on a daily basis, yet she didn't believe them, she was in essence calling him a liar.

Gail was dumbfounded by this and experienced enormous internal conflict: she knew her husband was not a liar, yet her low self-esteem would not allow her to believe the compliments he gave her. We asked Gail whether she would ever intentionally be unkind to her husband. She said, 'Never.' We then explained that whenever her husband gave her a compliment and she didn't believe him, she was being disrespectful. After all, a compliment is like being given a gift – her husband wanted his wife to know how beautiful, amazing and exceptional she was – and although we understood how difficult it might be for her to accept it, we told her that all she had to do was politely say thank you. This simple, kind act would start a new habit and help build her self-esteem.

Gail said that we were right and that she had never considered that before. She said she would never disrespect her beautiful husband again, and whenever he gave her a compliment, even if she found it difficult to accept as true, she would now say thank you in return. She accepted that he would never lie to her, and that it was wrong for her to be bad mannered and reject his compliment.

Finally, we talked about Gail's work. It was evident that, like many people with low self-esteem, she believed that she had got the job out of luck rather than merit. When we spoke to her about why she stayed in the role within her company when she was being bullied and wasn't happy, Gail said that she enjoyed her job and was really lucky to get it. We pointed out to Gail that nobody pays someone a salary if they are not capable of fulfilling the role, so we then asked her how many disciplinaries she had had. Gail replied, 'None.' We asked her how many times she had been told that she had not been doing the job properly, and again – other than the unpleasant comments from her manager about needing to do things faster, as she was being too friendly and talking too much with the elderly residents and their families – she said none. She went on to say that some remarks had been made about her appearance, things she had eaten and what she was wearing, and that she had been teased for something she had said, but Gail agreed that nothing had ever been said about the standard of her work.

She admitted that, in fact, she thought she went above and beyond what was needed in her job. We asked whether she had been interviewed before she was given the job, and Gail confirmed that she had been interviewed twice. The first time was by her manager, and the second time was by two senior members of the company who were above her manager. We asked Gail whether she thought the people who had conducted her second interview were fools. Gail replied, 'No.' We asked Gail why she thought they chose her. Gail looked up and laughed, and said, 'You've got me.' She joked, 'You two are good.' We had backed Gail into a corner. She had no other option but to see that she had got her job entirely on merit. We had provided her with overwhelming evidence that was contrary to what she had previously believed, so as to condition her inaccurate and destructive schema. She could not offer any evidence whatsoever that she wasn't good enough for the job.

To conclude our session, we asked Gail to look in the mirror and helped her to see herself through the eyes of someone who loved her unconditionally. (We share our Mirror Technique in Chapter 8, page 148.) When Gail opened her eyes and saw herself anew for the first time, she was able to see what everybody else saw. She looked at herself and said, 'I do need to lose a little bit of weight, but even if I didn't, I am not at all bad.'

Gail confirmed that she felt so much better about herself. She told us that she had a nice personality and a pretty face, that she was an achiever, having brought three children up on her own, and that, despite the challenges in her life, she had a good job, three children who adored her and a husband who loved her. We told Gail that we believed we had dealt with the block in her ability to lose weight, and hoped that now she could see how deserving she actually was, she would realise that she had never, ever failed.

The last time Gail contacted us, she had lost 4 stone (56lb/25kg) in weight. She was happier in work, and had spoken with her manager, which, although it was still not perfect, had drastically improved their relationship. Her email concluded that, in hindsight, she was glad that her first husband had cheated, because it has allowed her to meet her true soulmate.

In sharing Gail's story, and many other case studies of those we have helped, we hope we can inspire you to realise that you are exceptional, too, and that the key to your healthy life transformation could be within the pages of this book.

'You don't have to see the whole staircase, just take the first step.'

Martin Luther King Jr

In the next chapter, together we will start to analyse your timeline and work through your questionnaire to help you explain your eating patterns, locate the possible causes of your struggles with weight loss and identify the schemas that are driving your behaviour and potentially sabotaging your slimming success.

Wow! Two years ago with the Speakmans, and how my life has changed since then! Five stone gone [70lb/32kg], no fear of dogs, no more chocolate!

Michelle H.

5

Overeating

Eating and food were everything to me. Growing up, food dominated my life. Despite my mum having an eating disorder, she was a feeder. She cooked, she baked, and I could see her genuine pleasure if I, my dad and my siblings enjoyed her culinary delights. I was a people pleaser. I loved seeing my mum happy so would eat everything she gave me and would even ask for seconds, just to show her how much I appreciated her cooking.

Seeing Mum happy made me happy. I hadn't realised until seeing the Speakmans that, in an effort to still please my mum, I was eating and eating and eating, and had never switched that off!

Nik and Eva helped me to find the origin of my overeating, and once I'd addressed the fact that I was no longer living with my mum, my mum was no longer cooking my meals and that today the best way to make my mum happy is to spend quality time with her, it was like I had been given permission to stop overeating. Quite a revelation. Something so small had created such a big issue. It's great to no longer feel consumed by food, and to eat just when I'm hungry. From the bottom of my heart, thanks so much.

Angela L.

It's now time to take action, and to start addressing your behavioural patterns and your relationship with food.

Many of our clients have commented that we are like detectives, dissecting the information they have shared in their questionnaires and timeline. When helping people with weight issues, we also ask that they complete a food diary for a minimum of two (or ideally three) weeks, so as to document how they eat, when they eat and what they eat (this includes eating and drinking – essentially everything they put in their mouth). We are now going to ask you to do the same.

You can either use your own notebook, or take a photograph of our food diary on pages 78–79 and print it onto an A4 sheet. Slip your food diary into a plastic folder and keep it with you at all times. If you're at home, then leave it in the kitchen. If you are going out, place it in your pocket or handbag. If you're at work, keep it on your desk, and if you're on a car journey, leave it on the front seat.

It is important that you note down everything you eat and everything you drink, and also the time of day. We want you to start completing this food diary with immediate effect.

Food Diary

Keeping a food diary has many benefits. Documenting what you are eating makes you consciously aware of what you are consuming, and also accountable. Many of us eat unconsciously and without consideration, and can pop a biscuit, a bit of chocolate or a snack in our mouth at work or in the kitchen at home without even noticing. Such habitual behaviour is a pattern we are swept up in, and it is only when we take conscious action that we can interrupt that habit and start to make changes.

Writing down what you eat is also a great motivator in

helping you to avoid unhealthy food and make wiser choices. After reading our book, you may want to continue to keep a food diary, whether it's in a notebook, on our version or even using voice notes on your phone. Many people we have worked with have maintained their food diary as an ongoing support structure, with some moving on to doing it just from Monday to Friday, with weekends off, to keep themselves focused and in control. Perhaps you could consider doing this, too.

There are so many marketing companies trying manipulate your food intake, with a plethora of calorific temptations on every street corner, in every shop and magazine and on every channel on television. There is an abundance of food-orientated products, TV shows and advertisements poking at us, reminding us to eat, eat, eat.

However, there is only one person who will be with you 24 hours a day, seven days a week, for the rest of your life, and that person is you! Life is not only about living as long as possible, but also being in a fit state to enjoy it. You owe it to your future self, therefore, to be in control of how and what you eat, and writing your food diary is a big step towards that.

Substitutes

Eating is fun and central to most social gatherings. Sharing food is part of our evolution, and its role has been well documented throughout history. For example, evidence was found in a cave near Tel Aviv of meals prepared at a 300,000-year-old hearth where diners gathered to eat together.[17]

The symbolic breaking of bread together is at least as old as the Bible; therefore eating for pleasure and eating socially, to celebrate or unite people, is a part of who we are and what we do. In today's society, however, there is a big difference. Food is now abundant and an easily obtainable form of self-medication and short-term satisfaction. Furthermore, many foods have now been enhanced with sugars, fats, flavourings and additives, such as monosodium glutamate (MSG), which make your food seem tastier and increase your desire to keep eating. MSG is a food marketer's dream, as it blocks the messages to your brain that would normally let you know that you are full, encouraging you to eat more.

One study has shown that giving MSG to rats made them eat 40 per cent more than normal,[18] so if the food industry has that kind of power over your eating habits, is it any surprise that we live in an ever growing obese world?

Please be assured, however, that to be fit and healthy and to lose weight does not have to be about plates of leaves and tiny portions. Better choices and healthier substitutes are far more beneficial to you physically and mentally than restriction, which can often lead to eating obsessions, overeating and bingeing.

In Chapter 13 we will share numerous alternatives with you (see page 244), but first, we would like you to look at your food diary and either highlight or mark with an asterisk all the foods that you know sabotage your slimming success.

Behavioural Patterns

You are now starting to develop an informed, conscious awareness of what you are eating and how you can eat better, but your behavioural patterns around food are also of paramount importance to the success of your weight-loss journey.

Understanding when you eat, how you eat, and where you are, who you are with, what you are thinking, what you are feeling and what kind of a day you have had when you eat will all help you to find where issues may exist, and therefore what may need to be addressed to help your weight loss.

If you do not eat at regular intervals throughout the day, this can cause your blood sugar levels to drop, which can then lead to cravings of unhealthy carbohydrates for a quick rush of energy or to late-night binge-eating.

Look at your food diary and make a note of the spaces of time between when you eat. Make sure you consider the period of time from when you wake up to your first meal, too. Breakfast is what we have to 'break the fast' through the night.

As long periods without food contribute to overeating, if the length of time you are not eating in your waking hours exceeds four hours, you should consider setting an alarm or a reminder to have a bite to eat. Although this will require effort to begin with, you will start to create new habits if you persevere.

Options Available

Look at your food diary and all the unhealthy vice foods you have marked with an asterisk. If these items have been eaten while at home, remember that you can only eat what is available in your kitchen cupboards. Which is why we would like to help you construct a regular shopping list of groceries that will do you good rather than harm (see page 244).

Just as in life, if you do not plan for yourself, you will become a part of someone else's plan, and the strategically placed temptations in store when you shop are part of the supermarket chains' plans for bigger profits. We have all been in that situation where we go into a shop or supermarket for one or two things and walk out with a basket full of treats we had no intention of buying, often having forgotten what we went in for in the first place.

	Monday	Tuesday	Wednesday
breakfast			
morning			
mid-morning			
late-morning			
lunch			
afternoon			
mid-afternoon			
late-afternoon			
dinner			
evening			
late-evening			

Thursday	Friday	Saturday	Sunday

With that in mind, having a blueprint list of sensible groceries will support you as you shop and healthier choices will seem easier to make. Even better, if you shop online, you can use the same list of groceries and avoid the in-store temptations altogether.

Hydration

We have always been advocates of drinking lots of water and would recommend making a habit of it. Look at your food diary and evaluate how much you drink. Although the suggestion of drinking a minimum of eight glasses of water a day has been generally accepted, this amount does not take your height, weight and lifestyle into consideration. The research we have undertaken ourselves over the years suggests the more accurate equation of drinking a minimum of 0.6fl oz (17ml) of water per pound of your body weight. This figure is an absolute minimum to ensure that you are hydrated, which allows your body and organs to work efficiently.

The numerous benefits of drinking water are often overlooked – one of which is that it can help you lose weight. Interestingly, a study was undertaken in 2008 involving a group of overweight women over a 12-month period that supports this. Making no other lifestyle change at all, other than drinking more water, the women lost 4.4lb (2kg) of weight. The study also showed that approximately 17,000 calories were burned by each participant just from drinking extra water over that 12-month period. Additional calories are also burned if the water is cold, because the body uses up calories as it warms the water to body temperature.[19]

Finally, if that is not enough to convince you that drinking more water is a simple, cost-free and effective tool to help you win at weight loss, please also consider that dehydration can make you believe that you are hungry when you are not, therefore tricking you into eating more than you need (see page 61).

CASE STUDY
Brenda: Evening Binge-eater

Many people have shared their life stories with us over the years, both good and bad. However, when we met Brenda, we were both shocked by what she had endured – and touched by her bravery.

Brenda was from South America and had come to England for a 12-month work contract, during which she had made the decision to finally lose weight and address her binge-eating.

Brenda was approaching retirement and was very aware of the fact that her health was deteriorating as a consequence of her weight gain. However, despite trying numerous diets, going to see her doctor, speaking to a nutritionist at her health centre and having the best will in the world, Brenda could not maintain control of her eating. She just could not stop eating sugary snacks, particularly biscuits. She told us that, during her working day, she could quite happily go without eating anything, and was not at all tempted by her favourite sweet snacks, but the moment she returned home, had her evening meal and sat down, she was unable to have one or two biscuits with a cup of tea. Once she opened a packet of biscuits, she could not stop; she would have to eat the whole packet and often a second packet after that.

The next day Brenda would wake up feeling angry, ashamed and incredibly disappointed in herself. She would always promise herself that, to compensate for her excess, she would have just a little bit of fruit after her next evening meal, but every evening her plans would fall apart. She would cave in and again find herself stuffing empty biscuit packets in the bin, feeling as bad about what she had done as she had the previous evening.

We explained to Brenda that she was displaying a behaviour that in our opinion had a cause behind it, and that a positive intent may have started it, even if that positive intent is long in the past and no longer applies.

We asked Brenda to share a little of her life story with us, so we could find out when her binge-eating started. What had happened just prior to her being aware of it? What had been going on in her life?

Brenda went on to tell us that she had been married for 15 years and her husband had always liked to gamble. When she was in her late forties, she noticed that he had started to behave differently. He became distant and snappy and was rarely at home.

Brenda was absolutely shocked to the core when her husband one day just left without trace. He had taken some of his belongings and a few items of value and left her a note to say he was not coming back and that their marriage was over. Unbeknown to Brenda, her husband had built up a lot of debt, and had taken out a second mortgage on their home, which left the house in negative equity and Brenda unable to maintain the finances. Her house was eventually repossessed by the bank, and Brenda became homeless. She ended up sleeping in her car, with her few remaining belongings.

With no siblings, close family or parents alive, Brenda felt very alone. She did not want to burden her friends, and felt embarrassed and ashamed of where her life was at.

When she was then made redundant from her part-time job, she had no option but to live on the streets, which, for her, was terrifying. As she told us her story, we all became very sad and emotional, but we noted that Brenda frequently repeated the words, 'The person who was meant to protect and provide for me let me down. He stood and made a promise in church to all our friends and family, till death do us part, but he let me down.'

Now that she was homeless, there were many days when Brenda did not eat at all. She was visibly embarrassed when she told us that she had been so hungry that she had often eaten from bins. She went on to say that there were times when nothing passed her lips in a 24-hour period, or maybe more. Sometime later, Brenda was mortified when she was spotted by an old friend. Her friend embraced Brenda and cried from sadness, as well as relief that her dear friend was alive, as she had been so worried about her.

Brenda shared with her friend what had happened, apologised for not being in touch but explained that she had not wanted to burden her friends. She went on to share how embarrassed and ashamed she was, and how very let down she had been by her husband. Her friend immediately insisted that Brenda come home with her and stay until she got back on her feet.

When she got to her friend's home, Brenda was ravenously hungry, and she recalled her friend grabbing crackers, cheese, chocolate and biscuits the moment they walked through the door, and encouraging her to eat as much as she wanted. Brenda vividly remembers that she ate one biscuit after another, her tummy feeling fuller by the second, and for the first time in a long time she felt reassured, warm, fulfilled and safe. However, from that moment on, Brenda also developed a very unhealthy relationship with food, and with biscuits in particular.

Brenda had created two schemas while in a heightened emotional state:

Schema 1: Eating biscuits gives a feeling of safety and security.

Schema 2: Famine may occur at any moment, so when food is available I must eat to excess, as I do not know when my next meal is coming.

As a consequence of those two schemas, Brenda had started to eat to feel safe. Her positive intent was to protect herself from famine. Although during the day she was distracted by work, often not having time to eat, once she got home from work and ate her evening meal alone, she would feel lonely and insecure.

Brenda had never considered or addressed the schemas associated with her past, so we went on to ask her a few questions: 'When your friend came to your rescue and took you home, was it the biscuits that gave you the feeling of security?' Brenda asked us what we meant by this. We asked: 'What was it that actually gave you the feeling of security in that moment?'

Brenda replied, 'Well, I guess it was my friend.'

We expanded on our questions and pointed out that it was her friend, not the biscuits, that had put a roof over her head, given her meals, helped her find a job and got her back on her feet. We asked why she was crediting biscuits with what her friend had done. Surely this was disrespectful to her friend? After all, it wasn't biscuits who took her from the park bench to a cosy home.

Brenda immediately responded that she had never thought of it like that before, and that we were absolutely right – the feeling of security was down to her friend, not the biscuits. She agreed it was very disrespectful and unfair of her to credit biscuits, which were actually making her miserable. She said she now felt angry towards the biscuits, as they had been irrelevant to her turning a corner in her life after her husband left.

The moment Brenda said that she 'had never looked at it like that before', we knew that her perspective had changed. And once that happens, your thoughts, feelings and behaviours change, too.

We went on to address Brenda's second schema, which was protecting her from the famine she had experienced while she was homeless. Having gone for periods of time without eating, not knowing where her next meal was coming from, Brenda was bingeing 'just in case'. In essence, she was protecting her chances of survival.

We asked Brenda to repeat how she had managed to get into the situation of being homeless. Was it her decision? Was it her doing? Or might it have been as a result of an external factor or a third party?

Brenda confirmed that it was because of her husband. We asked her to elaborate. She added: 'Because my ex-husband took away my security, because he was my provider and he left me. He didn't provide for me and I lost everything.' We then asked Brenda whether she was still reliant on her ex-husband to provide for her? She replied, 'Absolutely not.'

We told Brenda that we understood that her ex-husband had been her provider in the past, and that, as a provider, he had let her down. We then asked her: 'Who is in sole charge of your life today, and will be for the rest of your life? Who is your provider now?'

Brenda went quiet. It was evident that she was considering everything we had put to her. She spoke softly at first, and then said with strength and authority: 'Just me. There is only me that I am relying on.'

We therefore asked the question: 'Brenda, are you ever going to let yourself down? Have you ever let yourself down?'

She said, 'I never have and I never will.' Brenda told us that as she was now working full time, she had a pension and savings. She concluded: 'I know I am going to be secure for the rest of my life, because I've made sure of that.'

When we pointed out to Brenda that as she had put money aside for a rainy day, she therefore did not need to eat excessively in case of a rainy day, we witnessed a very obvious visual shift in her physiology and her attitude.

Brenda contacted us some months later to let us know how drastically her eating patterns had changed. She was still quite flabbergasted that events from her past had caused her to binge-eat. She added that she now felt in control, and that the biggest shock to her was that she was even able to eat a biscuit or two without feeling compelled to finish the entire packet.

Your Healthy Life

1 Write a food diary for a minimum of two weeks, preferably three.

2 Note with an asterisk or highlight all the foods you know sabotage your slimming success.

3 Consider what alternatives or substitutions you could use for all the foods that are highlighted or marked with an asterisk.

4 Start to create a shopping list based on your healthier alternatives or substitutions (see page 243).

5 Use a different-coloured highlighter pen to mark the healthy choices on your food diary. To encourage your consumption of these healthy choices, add them to your shopping list.

6 Consider the times of day that you eat.

7 Consider what you are thinking and feeling, particularly when you overeat. What kind of day have you had?

Who have you interacted with? Did you get a good night's sleep?

8 Monitor your fluid intake, particularly water. Are you drinking enough? Invest in a reusable water bottle. Carry it with you, keep it close and sip water regularly.

9 Ensure you are getting enough sleep. Avoid getting overtired or sleep-deprived.

10 Address the cause of your unhealthy eating (see Chapter 6, page 92).

6

Emotional Overeating

Hi Nik and Eva. You have changed my life. I'm so grateful for what you have both done for me . . . I'm living my life now and I'm hopeful about the future. I've lost weight and I'm on my way to achieving two of my goals of gaining a counselling qualification and taking part in the London Marathon. Thank you to your team, Liv and Hunter for being so compassionate on the day. It made it so special. Thanks for everything.

Melissa

In this chapter we will look at the causes of emotional overeating and help you look at the questionnaire and timeline that you completed in Chapter 1, in order to identify and address the possible causes behind your emotional eating.

Identifying Emotional Eating

Emotional hunger comes on suddenly and usually creates a craving for junk food or sugary snacks, which will give an instant rush. It often feels impossible to overpower the urge, and leads to mindlessly eating high volumes of unhealthy food.

Unlike with normal hunger, when you are eating emotionally, you still find yourself needing to pick at food, even when you feel full. Emotional eating usually concludes with feelings of discomfort and bloating, followed by feelings of embarrassment, guilt and shame. Emotional hunger does not relent, and you find yourself focusing on specific foods, tastes and textures.

We will now share some case studies of people we have helped, in the hope that their stories might resonate with you and inspire you to challenge and positively condition the behavioural schemas that negatively impact your relationship with food.

Your body is the only vehicle you have to transport you through your life. Buckle up for an insightful journey, during which we hope you will discover why you overeat and find various ways to challenge your negative schemas and change your habits.

Common Causes of Emotional Eating

- **Self-medicating**
- **Protection**
- **Comfort**
- **Being in love/seeking a substitute for love**
- **Distraction**
- **Emulation/needing to belong**
- **Heartbreak/grief**
- **Self-sabotage**
- **Bullying**

Self-medicating

The need to self-medicate can arise as a consequence of numerous issues. If we experience painful, stressful, upsetting events, such as a relationship break-up, grief or some other form of loss, we may turn to food as a short-term comfort or distraction. Unresolved issues from the past that continue to cause emotional pain can similarly lead to self-medicating, as can feeling unloved, undervalued and not good enough or having rock-bottom self-esteem from being bullied or mistreated.

Food we enjoy helps to release feel-good hormones, which boost our mood. As endorphins are released, the pulse speeds up and we experience positive feelings, similar to when we fall in love. For most, food is easily accessible, and it can offer immediate relief and happiness, hence why so many turn to it for a quick fix.

Protection

In Chapter 7 (see page 124) you will read the case study of a lady who, as a child, felt she needed to be big in order to be able to physically protect herself. However, in some people, the need for protection may be more of an emotional need, and can stem from something less obvious, just as in Patrick's case.

CASE STUDY
Patrick: Protection

When we met Patrick, he was clinically obese. He was suffering with high-blood pressure, diabetes and sleep apnoea, which is characterised by pauses in breathing or periods of shallow breathing during sleep. Due to his sleep apnoea, every night he would have to connect himself to a very noisy machine with a face mask to ensure he didn't stop breathing during his sleep.

Patrick wanted to speak to us because he believed he had tried every diet on the planet. He felt he could answer any question about any diet or healthy-eating programme, because he had researched and tried them all. Yet despite that, after many years, he was still clinically obese and slowly gaining more and more weight. As we do with everybody we see, we asked Patrick to complete a questionnaire and also to look in a mirror and describe what he saw. The words he used were 'unattractive', 'fat' and 'ugly', which made us believe that his issues were linked to image, and there had to be good reason behind that.

What we learnt from the questionnaire was that Patrick's father had died when Patrick was a teenager, resulting in him stepping into his father's shoes and becoming entirely responsible for looking after his mum. He became the man of the house, and as a consequence of that, he devoted his life to his mum. It was also apparent from the questionnaire that Patrick's sexuality was ambiguous; he gave subtle hints that he had never been in a relationship, had never been in love and was lonely.

As we felt that 'attractiveness' was somehow key to Patrick's weight issues, we spoke to him at length about this. Eventually, he reluctantly mentioned that he might be bisexual, and after further discussion we established that Patrick believed there was a stigma attached to being gay. His parents had been born in a different era, and although he had never spoken to his mum about his sexuality, he thought she would find it incredibly difficult to understand if he were gay.

When we asked Patrick how he felt about speaking to his mum about this, he replied that he did not feel it was a subject he was comfortable discussing with her, which we completely understood. Unfortunately, he felt the topic of his sexuality would have to remain taboo.

Knowing that everything starts with a thought and that behind every behaviour there is a positive intent, we asked Patrick what the positive intent behind his weight might be. Patrick was unsure, so we suggested that perhaps, in view of what he had told us about his mum and his sexuality, he was sabotaging his own weight loss in an effort to make himself unattractive, thereby preventing himself from meeting anyone and having to face his predicament with his mum. 'Is it possible,' we suggested, 'that what you are actually doing is protecting yourself from having anyone fall in love with you, because the consequences of that could be painful for you?'

Patrick became very upset. He started to cry and said it was the first time he had ever allowed himself to admit this. He confirmed that his weight was his way of not having to face being open and honest with himself or his mum, because he loved his mum dearly and did not want to upset her. He was hiding behind his size.

We asked Patrick to consider speaking to his siblings and coming out to them as a starting point. Then, with their help, he could speak to his mum at a later date. He thought about it and told us that, because his mum was elderly and sick, he did not think now was the right time.

We had to be very open with Patrick and explain that we could help him build up his self-esteem and confidence, but that until he could be true to himself, he was likely to continue to self-sabotage and use food as a source of comfort and protection.

Patrick explained that he felt a lot of relief now that he could understand and acknowledge the reason behind his inability to maintain a healthy weight. It had provided an explanation and the realisation that he was not greedy or out of control. After helping him to accept that he had nothing to be ashamed of, and that his family would love him unconditionally no matter who he chose to love, he said he felt ready to start dropping little hints to his siblings, who he felt would be understanding.

Although we could not fix Patrick's situation fully due to his situation with his mum, he had found peace and begun his journey towards acceptance and self-love, which was an incredible start.

Survival is our primary instinct. In the modern world, we perceive thriving as surviving.

CASE STUDY
Melisa: Protection

We met Melisa on one of our trips to Los Angeles. Melisa was an actress and was fascinated with our work and philosophy. She was particularly interested in our view that all negative behaviours are symptoms, behind which lies a cause.

Excited to be 'analysed', Melisa shared that her negative behaviour was overeating. She went on to say, 'I think it could hold me back in my work as an actress, but I just can't stop.' She said that she tried so hard, yet she could not stop herself from giving in to what seemed like every possible temptation. We asked some questions about her life, looking to discover the key period when she started to gain weight. Melisa told us her story – that she had finished acting school and then become a waitress in order to survive between auditions. She said she went on a multitude of auditions without any success at all.

In her own words, she was a 'wholesome girl' and never skinny, but certainly she was not as big as she was now. The constant rejection from the auditions, however, had really started to take their toll on her. When Melisa had first started going to auditions, she had gone in with enthusiasm and excitement, but as time went on she started to attend them with a more negative attitude, as she now expected not to get the role. After every 'no', she would feel low and console herself with food, and punish herself with food for not being good enough. She said that it gave her a short-term, feel-good boost, particularly as she had a very sweet tooth. But as her size started to increase, the opportunities for auditions became fewer and fewer.

Then one day her agent told her that he had managed to secure her an audition for a theatre production, and his words were, 'I think you will be perfect for the part because they are looking for a big girl.' When she heard this comment, Melisa realised for the first time that she had gained an unacceptable amount of weight. Prior to this, she had tried to ignore it and wore baggy clothes in an effort to hide the extra pounds – obviously, she now realised, without success.

Still, Melisa went to the 'big girl' audition, and sure enough, when they told her about the role they added that they were looking for a big lady. Poor Melisa did not know whether to be offended by that or to play up to the part. So in that moment, she created the persona of a very confident and vivacious big woman, as she desperately needed this job. Two weeks later, she was recalled for a second audition, and then she was absolutely ecstatic to be told that she had got the part. This was a big turning point in Melisa's career. It was the first time she had secured a significant role, one that would offer her financial security for many months to come.

Melisa went on the road with the cast and enjoyed the new 'big girl' persona that she had created for herself. She laughed when she went out for dinner with her colleagues and they made comments such as, 'It's so unfair, we have to be really careful about what we eat', while Melisa would joke about how lucky she was that she could eat whatever she wanted.

Teasing herself and others about food now became a habit. She would say things like, 'Oh, if you are going to leave that, I will have it', and would continue to make jokes at her own expense to deflect attention from the fact that she had become something that she was not familiar or entirely happy with. After the production had concluded, Melisa continued to gain weight, and due to her now-known acting prowess, she was lucky to secure a second role, again as a 'big girl'.

When we were talking to Melisa she told us she did not need to be quite as big as she was. She said that she was now accepted as she was, and thought she had created a habit of eating large amounts of food. She admitted she could not stop and went on to say how she would hide food in her dressing room, house, handbag or car, and just felt she had to have lots of food around her at all times.

We asked Melisa what she thought it was that had got her that first role, having been for lots of unsuccessful auditions, and she replied, 'My size.' We immediately knew that her response was the answer to her weight problem.

We then said, 'So what you are saying is that, even if you were a useless actress, you would still have got the part, as it was your size that impressed them.'

Tears started to form in Melisa's eyes. She replied, 'I had failed so many auditions, I genuinely believed I was a useless actress.'

Although our point – that she had attributed her success to the wrong thing – was now starting to filter through, to extinguish any other excuses she may have tried to sell herself, we also asked: 'Did you get the role because no one else had applied for the role?' Melisa laughed and admitted that there were in fact lots of other people going in after her at the audition, as she remembers seeing them in the waiting area.

We asked her to tell us what that meant about her and her acting ability. Melisa's face lit up as she said, 'They wanted me because I ticked all their boxes.'

As we chatted with Melisa, we pointed out that her positive intent, which had led her to create the schema that was standing in the way of her being able to lose weight, was: 'Being big keeps me in work.'

Being entirely self-reliant financially, it was no wonder that the thought of losing weight might feel catastrophic for Melisa. Her inaccurate schema was that being big was keeping a roof over her head, and therefore to protect herself and her livelihood, she believed she had to be big.

We asked Melisa if she wanted to lose weight and she confirmed that she did. We asked her to tell us why she wanted to lose weight, and her answer was that she was worried about her health. We asked her how being healthy would impact her livelihood, and she replied, 'I do feel I have another string to my bow being a bigger girl, as there are fewer actresses in big-girl roles, and more importantly, there are fewer actresses with a CV that highlights their capability in the role.' So despite her fears for her health, Melisa clearly believed that being slimmer might damage her career.

Knowing that survival is our primary instinct, and that earning a living contributed to Melisa's survival, we pointed out that she now had a choice. She had it in her power to lose weight if she wanted to, though it might prove detrimental to her career. We also advised her that we could not change her primal instincts, and that at this stage she would likely fight against any potential weight loss if she believed that her size helped her get better roles.

She thought about this and confirmed that it was not the right time for her to lose a significant amount of weight, but that, in the future, if she were to meet somebody and find added financial security, she would then be able to consider losing weight and going for different kinds of acting roles.

We felt a little sad that Melisa felt trapped in this way, wanting to lose weight yet feeling unable to do so, but equally, she now had an answer to her weight issues and could change her terminology from 'I can't lose weight' to 'I can lose weight when I want to, but I choose not to right now.'

We also pointed out that even though she was overweight, this did not mean she had to be unhealthy, and suggested that she start going to the gym, exercising, walking more and making healthier dietary choices. She agreed and felt very excited that she could become healthier and lose some weight, yet remain in the bracket she deemed necessary for the 'big girl' roles.

We have met up with Melisa on subsequent trips, and she told us that whereas before she felt she was on a downward spiral of destruction from just eating and eating, she now felt healthier and more in control, particularly because we had pointed out that she could be big and healthy. This had significantly altered her mindset, as had the realisation that it was her acting skills, not her size, that were key to her success as an actress.

Are You Protecting Yourself?

We would now like you to look at your timeline and the answers you gave in your questionaire.

* **Has anything occurred in your life that might have led you to use weight as a form of protection?**

* **Did you need to be big to stop people loving you because that could lead to emotional pain?**

* **Did you need to be big to hide away and not be seen?**

* Did you need to be physically big to protect yourself from someone?

* Is being big part of your persona, which you fear losing?

* Is being big a benefit to you socially?

* Is being big a benefit to your work?

If any of these apply to you, in Chapter 12 we will share suggestions to help you address and positively condition these schemas.

Need for Comfort, Love, Distraction, Grief or Heartbreak

We will often see in a movie or sitcom someone easing a broken heart with a tub of ice cream. The truth is that, in real life too, eating can be a brief distraction that temporarily silences uncomfortable or unpleasant emotions, such as loneliness, fear, sadness, anxiety, heartbreak, grief, resentment and shame. For many, food becomes the plaster used to try to cover the wound.

As tasty food can stimulate the release of the 'feel-good hormone' dopamine, it can offer us comfort when we're feeling sad, lonely or in need of a little love. Furthermore, research suggests that we actually get two hits of this 'feel-good hormone' when we eat, as the dopamine release in the brain occurs at two different times – when we first ingest the food, and again when it reaches the stomach.[20]

We would now like to share Ruby's story with you.

CASE STUDY
Ruby: Grief/Distraction/Heartbreak

Ruby had never had an issue with weight throughout her life; she had always had a very normal relationship with food, eating just when she was hungry and never feeling concerned about her weight or what she was eating. However, when Ruby's husband became unwell and she began to look after him, as his health deteriorated, so did her eating patterns.

Ruby found herself eating more and gaining weight. But because she was so busy and distracted by nursing her sick husband, she didn't have time to think about her weight gain, so she pushed it to one side. Her husband was her priority, and so she became preoccupied with his care.

Sadly, Ruby lost her husband and contacted us 18 months after he had passed away, as she now found herself in a situation where she had reached a dangerous weight. Even more concerning to her was that she felt she had no control over her eating. She found herself in a vicious cycle, which was drastically hindering her ability to live her life, and was desperate for our help.

Ruby's situation is not uncommon; many people turn to food when they are grieving, and it is perfectly understandable. Eating releases dopamine, commonly referred to as the 'pleasure' chemical, which is linked to rewarding behaviour, and also serotonin, which contributes to feelings of well-being and happiness, so it is unsurprising that during these times of sadness, Ruby turned to food to help her feel better. In essence, she was self-medicating her grief with food. With that in mind, we knew that the best way to help Ruby was to address her feelings of grief. She also needed more positive, therapeutic distractions that could contribute to better stimulating the dopamine and serotonin neurotransmitters in her brain.

We began our session by addressing her issues around grief. Naturally, Ruby was heartbroken, but we helped her to realise that her husband's life had far more value than his death. Also, although we had complete sympathy for her loss and thoroughly understood her grief, we asked her to consider what her husband's course of action might have been had the roles been reversed. Ruby was confident that, despite being heartbroken, her husband would be getting on with his life – whereas she had put her life on hold. She also said that before he passed away, he had made her promise that she would not mope, and that she would live her life on behalf of them both.

She hadn't really appreciated his words until that moment, as she had been too consumed by his loss, and had never discussed this conversation since his passing. We highlighted that, despite her husband's physical absence, the memories she had of him would never leave her, and therefore her husband would always be a part of her life. He had had no choice about his life ending, we told her, but in his honour she could choose to live her life for them both, as he had requested, so that, through her, his memory could go on to experience her laughter, love, fun and adventures. We also pointed out that it was disrespectful to him not to celebrate his life and the life they'd had together. We asked if she was willing to do this for herself and her husband, and Ruby confirmed that she was. She agreed with us that she owed it to her husband to fulfil her promise to him.

Until she spoke with us, Ruby was very preoccupied with the period of time surrounding her husband's death, but the more she started to talk about him, the more she began to tell us stories – things she hadn't thought about for many years. These memories included the funny things he had done, the little tricks he had played on her, the romantic gestures he made, the wonderful holidays they had taken and the incredible memories they had made together. As we talked, there was a visible lift in Ruby and her shoulders started to relax. The happy memories of her husband were starting to filter through.

The next stage in Ruby's recovery was to look at how her life could move forward, and so we proceeded to a goal-setting session – an important element in the recovery from emotional eating.

We asked Ruby to consider all the things in her life that she had ever wanted to do, all the things she had ever wanted to see, experience, taste or say to someone, all the friends she wanted to make or reconnect with, all the hobbies she wanted to try or rekindle from the past. We asked her to consider what kinds of things she would regret never having done if this were her last day on earth. Once we had a list, we were then able to compartmentalise these into goals for one year, three years, five years, ten years and ten years plus into the future.

We suggested to Ruby that she work on just three of her one-year goals to start with. Once she had taken the first step towards one of them, she could move on to the next.

Finally, we shared suggestions of activities Ruby could undertake that are known to naturally stimulate our dopamine and serotonin neurotransmitters. These include activities such as hugging – she confirmed that she had lots of lovely family members whom she knew, if she were to visit them more often, would give her lots of hugs.

She also added that she had always wanted a little dog and knew she could get a lot of love and cuddles from a dog, so she added this as a one-year goal. It had been something she had put on hold when her husband became ill, so she was determined to action this as a priority.

We also highlighted that laughter is an amazing natural tool to help us feel better, so we suggested she start watching more comedies and things she found funny. She said she would; instead of sitting and eating in the evenings, she would now start watching boxsets of her favourite comedies. Finally, we also suggested exercise as another effective, natural stimulant of our feel-good hormones. We discussed which activities she enjoyed, and as she loved swimming, she confirmed that this would be easy to implement once or twice a week. This was an amazing idea because not only would it make her feel better, healthier and happier and give her something new to concentrate on, but it was also another opportunity to meet people and make new friends.

Ruby had a long journey ahead of her, but she left us feeling excited, as she now had so many things to look forward to and keep her occupied. We have taken great pleasure in observing Ruby's progress on social media. She has travelled, and her pictures are illuminated with the biggest, most beautiful smiles, which in turn has put the biggest smiles on our faces, too. We feel incredibly blessed and grateful to have made a difference in her life.

> *It's never too late to start living your life again.*

CASE STUDY
Bev: Need for Comfort and Love

Bev, a mum in full-time employment, asked for our help because she wanted to be more motivated to exercise and eat healthily. Prior to our appointment, we asked Bev to complete a food diary, a questionnaire and a timeline so that we could look for evidence, clues and patterns of behaviour.

What Bev told us was what that she had started to gain weight around the age of 10 or 11, although it had never been as bad as it was now. Bev believed things had got far worse as a consequence of her high-pressure job, having a family and not having time for herself.

We looked through Bev's food diary and highlighted the areas where she could substitute what she was eating for better, healthier options. We also found that her eating patterns were quite erratic, in that she would go for very long periods throughout her working day without eating, then later she would consume empty calories – foods containing sugar, simple carbohydrates and high fats, which she would grab from a shop close by, such as a petrol station – most likely for a quick boost of energy.

Bev would go on to eat a significant amount of food later in the evening, because by the time she got home, her energy levels had depleted, making her body feel as though it needed energy quickly, and so again she opted for quick-fix carbs.

It was also evident that Bev was going to bed far too late and not getting enough sleep, which was also contributing to her overeating, most likely as a consequence of the 'hunger hormone' known as ghrelin, the production of which accelerates when we're tired.

Looking at Bev's timeline, there were some things that stood out to us, particularly involving her mum. Bev shared that, although she was a lovely lady, her mum was a single parent and sadly an alcoholic. The consequence was that, as a little girl, Bev had experienced very little quality attention at home.

Bev had a much older sister who did not live with them, and therefore she had lived the life of an only child, which was incredibly lonely. Through our discussions, we established that her destructive eating patterns had started when she was a little girl in her bedroom. Her mum would often pick up treats and unhealthy snacks for Bev out of guilt, and would often say, 'I have bought you chocolates and sweets to cheer you up.'

In hindsight, Bev realised this was likely her mum's way of saying, 'I'm not around for you, but here is a substitute to show you that I care.' This led to Bev creating the schema that food equalled love, and therefore she would take her snacks into her bedroom, where she would sit alone, watching television and eating. She would console herself that her mum did love her, and that this was reflected in the treats she had bought for her.

As time wore on, whenever Bev was studying and alone, or whenever her relationships broke down, she would turn to food for solace and comfort – after all, to Bev food meant love.

We worked through the issues that we saw on Bev's timeline and helped her see that it wasn't food providing her with love; it was her perception that food was love.

We asked her to consider how food had helped her. She was lonely and wanted comfort, so had the food ever spoken with her? Cuddled her? Taken her somewhere? Made her laugh? We asked what she had wanted from her mum when she was a little girl. She confirmed that all she had ever really wanted was quality time with her mum and a hug. We asked if food had ever provided that. Bev responded, 'No, it never has.'

We then asked Bev how she showed her children that she loved them. She confirmed that she would never say to them, 'Here is a bar of chocolate', to substitute for the words 'I love you' – that would never suffice. She added, 'I say "I love you" and scoop them up for hugs. We spend quality time together. That means love to me, not food.' We had established that Bev's definition of love was quality time and physical contact, and that food had never offered her that, and this realisation had a significant impact on Bev. She laughed and said, 'That is so strange, I have never thought of it like that before.'

Having challenged and conditioned Bev's schema around food, we then moved on to a secondary issue that could be negatively affecting her ability to lose weight – her self-confidence.

The fact that her mum had been an alcoholic during Bev's childhood may have created the feeling that she wasn't good enough as a daughter. She may have thought that, had she been good enough, when she pleaded with her mum to stop drinking, her mum would have stopped. To help her find peace with this era of her life, we asked Bev to tell us a little more about her mum's life. Sadly, her mum had had a turbulent childhood and, in addition, had been in a violent marriage with Bev's father.

We asked Bev to consider that, just as she had self-medicated with food, her mum had self-medicated with alcohol because of her emotional pain, and that this was obviously not Bev's fault. This was a very emotional moment for Bev, as she acknowledged that, against the odds, her mum had done her very best.

We moved on to look at Bev's food diary and helped her to identify some small changes that could be made. This included ensuring that she ate something for breakfast, such as a healthy, dairy-free product from a local coffee shop that she knew would be available and easy to just grab on her way into the office. She volunteered the information that somebody always undertook a lunch run at work, and therefore she vowed that she would ask them to buy her a healthy salad every single day, and would pay them in advance, so that her salad appeared even if she did not ask for it.

In relation to exercise, Bev said that there was an aerobics studio below her office, and to help motivate her to go, we suggested it would be a great idea to get a few other work colleagues to join in, as the more people there were involved, the less likely she would be to quit. Having that group support would help. Bev also suggested that a charity angle would be another great motivator.

Some months later, Bev emailed to update us, saying that it was amazing how taking control of her personal life had given her a better quality of life and a better work ethic. She now had more energy and clarity at work, and more energy and enthusiasm to do fun and active things with her children. She was feeling healthier and fitter, and had consequently bought bikes for herself and her children – they were now going out on bike rides most weekends.

By making just a few small changes to her approach to eating and exercise, and by resolving the issues from her past, Bev had transformed her perspective and her life for the better.

Are You Eating to Comfort Yourself? Or Heal a Broken Heart?

* When did your relationship with eating change negatively? Look at your timeline. What was happening in your life around then?

* Have you ever felt you needed love or comfort? If so, when? Compare that with your timeline.

* Did you feel you lacked love as a child? If so, when and why? What was your relationship like with food then?

* Have you ever had your heart broken? How does that feel today? If you were to score the discomfort you feel when thinking about that now, what would it be out of ten? Discomfort of six or above is significant and needs to be addressed, as this could be a cause of your eating habits.

* Have you ever suffered the loss of a loved one? How does that feel today? If you were to score the discomfort thinking about that now, what would it be out of ten? Discomfort of six or above is significant and needs to be addressed, as this could be a cause of your eating habits.

In Chapter 12, we will share suggestions to help you address and positively alter and condition this schema.

Are You Emulating? Do You Have a Need to Belong?

We all like to belong, whether to a family or group of friends or work colleagues. Like pack animals, we find safety and an increased chance of survival in numbers.

We also put ourselves under great pressure to belong, as it tends to make life more fun. With popularity comes inflated status and 'street cred'. For some, particularly if they felt excluded in childhood, peer pressure and the desire to belong can lead them to compromise their standards, leading to actions that may be contrary to their personal values and beliefs.

> *People like people that are like themselves.*

The need to belong leads many to try their first cigarette or their first alcoholic drink. And to some degree we all manipulate our personality a little depending on the group of people we are with. You may have noticed that with some friends you become a little louder and more giddy, whereas with others you are more serious and sedate.

However, you may be surprised to learn that emulating others and wanting to belong could be a cause of your unwanted negative behaviours surrounding food.

CASE STUDY
Amy: Emulating

Amy was the youngest of four children and there was a significant age gap between her and her older siblings. By the time Amy was eight years of age, all of her siblings had married and moved away from home, leaving her at home with her parents. Then, when Amy was nine, her father also left the family home; he had been having an affair and, Amy learned, had had another daughter while still married to her mum. By the time the affair had come to light, he was ready to move abroad with his new family, leaving Amy and her mum at home alone.

This situation was devastating for both Amy and her mum, but Amy tried hard to be strong for her mum and would not allow her to see her cry. Despite this show of strength, Amy was heartbroken. She felt her father had not just left her mother, he had also abandoned his daughter, choosing his other family over her. She felt unhappy, worthless and not good enough. On the handful of trips she made to visit her father, she felt like an outsider, intruding on a family she did not know. Her father had become a stranger.

At this time, Amy's mum was already slightly overweight, but once Amy's dad had left, she started to put on weight at quite a fast pace. It continued to creep up, even into Amy's adult life and, according to Amy, her mother had never lost the weight.

After her dad left, Amy and her mum would sit in front of

the television and eat far more snacks and unhealthy food than they had ever eaten before. Amy's mum was depressed and therefore did not cook, so they lived off takeaway meals. Once Amy was in her twenties, she met somebody, married and had two children of her own. As her mum had never met anyone else after her dad, Amy stayed close to where her mum lived, because she felt that her mum needed her.

By the time Amy came to see us, she was clinically obese and was considering a gastric band, as she had been told by her doctor that she was at high risk of diabetes. She felt very unhealthy and unfit. As a devoted mum, Amy felt she needed to lose weight for the sake of her children.

Having spoken at length with Amy and having read through the questionnaire she had completed prior to our session, it was obvious that the weight gain had started when her dad left. Understandably, Amy had copied her mum's behaviour, and as a consequence she had gained weight at the same time. Amy's partner had never known her any other way, and therefore she had never really felt the need to lose weight until she'd had children.

We explained to Amy that people like people who are like themselves, and that Amy was still trying to emulate her mum to make her feel better. She had started this behaviour with good intentions but had never stopped.

We asked whether that felt right to Amy. She responded that she had never considered it, yet there was definitely truth in everything we had said. Even now, Amy would speak to her mum daily, and together they would chatter about their weight, dieting, treats and what they were going to cook for dinner, and therefore, whether positive or negative, the topic of food was common ground between them and undoubtedly gave them a closeness. Amy admitted that she did not really know what else she and her mum would talk about if it wasn't food.

However, now that Amy was aware that this was very

probably a contributing factor to her inability to lose weight, she felt it was something she needed to address. We pointed out that, whereas the current common ground between her and her mum was making them both unhealthy, would it not be better to instigate a new commonality that would encourage a healthier lifestyle for them both? We asked Amy if she loved her mum, and of course she answered yes. So we put it to Amy that if her intention was to care for her mum, would it not be more loving and caring to encourage her to be healthy? We recommended that Amy take her mum to a slimming club, health club or local leisure centre – a far more positive way to find common ground that would not only improve their health, but also constitute a social activity they could do together.

Amy thought that was an amazing idea and felt that if she were to encourage her mum, she would probably embrace the idea of joining a slimming club together.

After leaving us, Amy called her mum and was very open and honest about our session, telling her that she had realised that after her dad had left, they had both gained a lot of weight because they were comforting themselves with food. Now that she had children of her own, she explained, she felt it was important that she lose weight, but she didn't want to go on the journey alone – she wanted her mum to join her. Amy was surprised by how excited her mum was at the prospect of having something new to aim for together.

They talked more and Amy helped her mum to deal with the loss of her husband, which she and Amy had never really spoken about before; it had been a taboo subject. This gave them both the release they needed to set them free from a past that had been holding them back and making them very unhealthy.

We are very pleased to share that Amy and her mum have both now lost weight and have a far more positive and healthy relationship with food – and with each other.

Are You Emulating Someone in Order to Belong?

* Did a parent or close family member have a bad relationship with food and issues associated with repetitive dieting when you were growing up?

* Did someone you were very close to have a bad relationship with food and issues associated with repetitive dieting when you were growing up?

* Do you live, socialise or have regular contact with someone who also has issues around weight loss and overeating?

* Do you speak to someone regularly about food, weight loss, dieting? If so, who?

* Look at your timeline and questionnaire. Who features regularly or with significance? Consider their relationship with food and weight loss.

In Chapter 12, we will share suggestions to help you address and positively condition this schema.

Were You Bullied? Are You Self-sabotaging?

In our experience over the last 20-plus years, we have found that the most common cause of self-sabotage, low self-esteem and self-medicating is bullying. Those we have helped have been subjected to bullying at home, at school, at work and even within friendship circles.

The consequences of bullying in relation to overeating and weight gain can include:

1   Self-medicating with food to help ease emotional pain.

2   Giving up on diets, healthy-eating programmes and any self-improvement techniques due to a belief that you do not deserve to look and feel good.

3   Sabotaging your own slimming success in the belief that your efforts are futile, because you have been made to feel useless and a failure.

4   Sabotaging your efforts to lose weight as a form of self-punishment or self-loathing.

CASE STUDY
Katie: Bullying

Katie's story was something we had come across many, many times before. A working mum, in a happy marriage, Katie told us that despite a good life, her biggest issue was her inability to interact with her two young children at play areas and parks because of her size. She said that she did not have the energy to run, play and do things with them, and felt enormously guilty, as she would have to ask her sisters or husband to take the children out instead of her.

Katie made it very clear that she had no desire to be thin, she just wanted to be healthy. However, she could not maintain a diet or a fitness regime and therefore desperately needed our help.

We explained to Katie that there are four important elements to achieving a sustainably healthy weight: to eat healthily, to move more, to be aware of your environment and to address the cause behind your behaviour.

No one is born overweight, so we asked Katie to recall when there may have been a turning point in her life that caused her to overeat. Katie was adamant that she did not know; she had always been 'a big girl', she said, and could not recall ever being not overweight.

Before Katie's session we asked her to bring along some pictures of herself during her childhood, and when we looked through these photographs it was very evident that actually she wasn't overweight as a little girl. As Katie looked at the photographs in front of her, she was shocked to note that she was not fat at all. She had always considered herself to be 'a big girl', yet now, Katie described herself as looking like 'a pretty normal kid'. The photographic evidence could not be argued with, and we felt this was significant.

Looking at Katie's forms we could see that she had been bullied at school, so we asked her what kinds of things had been done or said to her. Katie said that the bullying had never been physical, and that it had taken the form of name calling. We asked what kinds of names she was called, and Katie said she was always called 'the big one' and 'honey monster'.

Armed with this information, we said to Katie, 'So you were always the big one in class. Is that correct?' Katie confirmed it was. Having seen her school photographs, we then asked her to explain where she stood in terms of height in the class, compared to the other children. Was she the tallest, the shortest or somewhere in between? Katie responded, 'I was always the tallest and always so much bigger than everyone else in the class.' This was our eureka moment; we had found the answer to Katie's ongoing problems with eating.

We asked Katie to tell us once more what people had said about her at school. She again replied, 'I'm the big one.' We asked her, if she were a little girl and had a group of friends of different sizes and ages, how would she refer to the eldest and tallest? Would she say they were the tall kids or the big kids? Katie's hands came up to her face and she said, 'The big kids! We called them the big kids because they were bigger than us.'

For the first time, Katie realised that she had completely misunderstood the situation. She had always believed that she was being bullied because she was the 'big one', thinking this meant fat, not tall, so she had fulfilled the title as she had perceived it. Katie accepted that children can look for differences that they can use to deflect attention from themselves, often due to their own insecurities. Therefore, for many children, name calling or the teasing of others can be used as form of protection, an element of 'tease or be teased' or 'bully or be bullied'. This misunderstanding of perception had made Katie feel bad about herself, which gave her low self-esteem and led to her self-sabotaging, so that, even when she tried to lose weight and do exercise, unconsciously she was telling herself, 'Well, what is the point? I'm the big one. I've always been the big one.'

This realisation meant a great deal to Katie. She cried as the burden of pain from all those years ago lifted.

After that, for the first time Katie found being fit and healthy not just easy, but also pleasurable. She told us that she had started to make small changes in her life that were making a significant difference. She walked her daughter to school and would then walk the longer route to work. Once she felt that her fitness levels had increased, she started to go to the gym.

Katie has become a fit, healthy mum and feels far more confident than she ever has before.

CASE STUDY
Jackie: Bullying and Self-medicating

When Jackie walked into our health club back in 2001, her posture gave away a lot. She walked in with her head stooped as if she did not want to be seen, and her shoulders were rounded as if they were carrying all the world's troubles. She clearly felt very uncomfortable, and looked as though she did not want anyone to see or look at her.

Back then, Jackie was a UK size 24, and when we sat and spoke with her, she started to tell us that she wanted to make changes in her life.

She was a mum, who worked in a canteen, serving food in a male-orientated industry. She had very low self-esteem and confidence, and as the weeks went by and we got to know her, she started to tell us a little bit more about her life. It transpired that Jackie was in a violent marriage, where she was often belittled and made to feel worthless and inadequate. She stayed because she didn't think she was capable of managing life on her own with her children. She went on to tell us that the abuse was not just within the four walls of her home, because at work, even though she knew it wasn't done with malice, the men would often tease her because of her size. When coming into the canteen they would say things like, 'Hope Jackie hasn't eaten all the chips.'

What her colleagues perceived as 'fun banter' was very hurtful to Jackie and, coupled with how she was being made to feel at home, it was further destroying her sense of self-worth.

We explained to Jackie the importance of understanding her eating patterns and the cause behind them, so we asked her to complete a food diary. It was evident that her eating was far worse just before lunchtime during the working week, and in the evenings, particularly around the time her children went to bed, on Thursdays, Fridays, Saturdays and Sundays. Together, we tried to figure out what the common denominator might be at these specific times, and Jackie had a lightbulb moment. She was absolutely sure that she would start to snack as lunchtime approached in order to 'cheer herself up', as she dreaded having to fake a smile at all the cutting comments during her lunch shift. The common link with her Thursday-to-Sunday-evening binges was that these were the nights when her husband would go to the pub and often come home drunk and aggressive. It was clear that Jackie was self-medicating. She felt bad, and food was distracting her from that fact and offering her a brief moment of comfort and respite.

Over the weeks and months, we started to talk to Jackie about the situation she was facing. It was important for her recovery that she understood why some people become bullies and that her husband's attacks were not her fault but due to his own issues and insecurities. Jackie needed to accept that she did not deserve to be treated as she was, and that there was no truth in the things that were being said to her.

Talking through these issues, we started to see a real change in Jackie. She was losing weight and becoming more confident, and it was a pleasure to watch her transformation.

Over the course of 12 months, Jackie went from a size 24 to a size 14, and one day, very proudly and confidently, she told us that she had left her husband. Because she had taken control of her health and started to think more about herself, she was now starting to flourish and be the person she was supposed to be. It was interesting to note that, as Jackie had started to lose weight, her ex-husband had become even more abusive.

Six months later, when we were at a social event, we saw a stunning, confident, size-12 woman walk into the room.

It was Jackie, and we felt overjoyed for her. Her life went on to change in numerous ways. She left her job and met somebody who loved and respected her, whom she married a few years later.

We have been so fortunate to see many people transform their lives by making one simple decision. Jackie's was to embrace our suggestions, and as a consequence, she changed her life entirely.

Have You Ever Been Bullied?

We would now like you to look at your timeline and the answers to your questionnaire.

* **Have you ever been bullied?**

* **Has anyone ever made you feel inferior or worthless, spoken down to you or been unkind to you?**

* **Have you ever felt intimidated by anyone?**

* **Has anyone ever called you names that still hurt your feelings when you think about it now?**

* **Is there anyone in your life now who makes you feel bad about yourself, undervalued or not good enough?**

* **Have you ever laughed off teasing comments in front of people but found them hurtful on the inside?**

In Chapter 12, we will share suggestions to help you address and positively alter this schema.

7

Overeating Due to Trauma

I can't ever thank you enough for everything you have done for me. I suffered for five years with PTSD after a road traffic accident and I never, ever thought I would have my life back . . . I'm now flourishing, have lost 96 per cent of my [excess] body weight and am doing far better than anyone expected. I am just so happy, and everyone around me is so happy for me.

Jo

We have found that negative emotions, anxieties and damaging behaviours are usually the consequence of having experienced some form of trauma. For example, phobias are often the result of having had or having witnessed a traumatic event. Low self-esteem is often symptomatic of bullying, while obsessive compulsive disorder (OCD) can be the residual effect of trauma during childhood, either at home or at school.

Overeating, food addiction, binge-eating and weight gain can also be the consequences of trauma – either prolonged or singular. Equally, post-traumatic stress disorder (PTSD) can be the culprit behind your issues with weight.

> **A new study provides further evidence of the link between psychological stress and weight gain, after finding that a woman's risk of obesity may be heightened by bad life experiences.**
>
> *Medical News Today*[21]

Research published in the journal *JAMA Psychiatry* found that women with post-traumatic stress disorder were more likely to be overweight or obese, and gained weight faster. They also found that people who are stressed crave unhealthy, high-calorie foods.[22] Therefore, in this chapter we would like to share with you case studies where trauma has proved to be a significant contributor to weight gain and the inability to lose weight. We will also share with you tips on how to address trauma, which should prove useful even if right now you are unaware of a trauma causing your weight gain but just know that carrying any negative emotional baggage does not serve you.

CASE STUDY
Ruth: Prolonged Trauma

When we met Ruth, she told us that in desperation to lose weight, she had tried everything. She had been on all the different diet plans, joined numerous gyms and booked in with numerous personal trainers. Despite her best efforts, however, she had struggled to maintain a healthy-eating plan, and as a consequence she felt bad about herself.

Given that seeking third-party advice wasn't helping her to lose weight, she decided to train and qualify as a fitness and aerobics instructor, and she then went on to achieve a degree and a masters in nutrition. She had been studying for years in a bid to find the answer to why, if she ever lost weight, she only ended up putting it back on – and more besides.

Ruth completed our thorough questionnaire and also a timeline, and we began by asking her to think back to memories of when she was happy with her weight. We then asked her to consider when she first became aware of her weight gain, or when others started to notice it. Ruth told us that it was in her early teenage years.

Looking through her timeline, we found two enormously significant events that occurred in her life around that time. The first was that she had been abused from childhood by a family member. Although she always despised what was happening, at the age of 11 or 12 she started to understand what it actually meant. The second significant event was that she also started to be severely bullied at school. She was introverted and shy, which she attributed to her homelife, and hoped that if she hid away, she might not be seen. She felt different, and did not want to let people in. The bullying was both physical and verbal, and Ruth described the primary bully as a big girl, both in height and weight, who was very imposing and quite frightening. Because the bully was a big girl, Ruth believed at the time that she must also be braver, and that people were so intimidated by her size that they did not stand up to her.

We went on to talk about the abuse Ruth had endured, particularly about how it had ended, which was towards the latter end of her bullying at school, when Ruth finally fought back against her abuser. Ruth started to eat more in her teens, and when she had gained weight and was bigger in size, the day eventually came when she felt able to say no and physically push her abuser off. The abuse then ended, and we explained to Ruth that this event had most likely created the schema: 'Being big keeps me safe.'

Ruth could not speak for some time as she processed this information. As she collected herself, she told us that she recalled having those thoughts, that being bigger would help her to 'fight him off'. She went on to say how she had locked that thought away and not revisited it, which we explained was common; when something is very painful, it is often easier to lock it away and not face it.

To help change the schemas that Ruth had created, we first established that the bullying at school was not personal to her. The girl was a bully who undoubtedly bullied other people, too. The fact that Ruth was withdrawn at school because of the abuse she was enduring made her a target. We also pointed out to Ruth that, by inspiring her to get bigger, the bully had played a role in helping Ruth to end the abuse, which was an unlikely positive to have come from that situation. Ruth agreed, and said the words we like to hear: 'I have never thought about it like that before.' Ruth then went on to share that the girl who had bullied her had had a challenging life herself, which was something everyone at the school was aware of.

We then talked about the abuse. We said to Ruth, 'You became big to keep yourself safe. Have you completed the task it was intended for?' Ruth confirmed that she had. We went on to ask: 'Do you still need protection? Do you still need to be big?' Ruth said no. We asked if the abuser was still a part of her life and Ruth again said no – her abuser had passed away. We concluded by asking whether she had ever needed to fight anyone else off. Ruth confirmed that the abuse had ended when she was 14, when she had gained the strength to physically stop it, and did not need to be big anymore to be safe.

It was evident that Ruth's mind was racing and that our conversation had resonated. It all made sense to her. She recalled a time when she had given herself a goal to lose weight in order to wear a UK size-12 red dress to a family party. Given that she had been a size 22 when she'd bought the dress, she'd had quite a journey ahead of her but felt this might motivate her, which it did. Ruth attained the size 12 and went to the party looking and feeling a million dollars.

She had been delighted with the way she looked, but she'd never understood why, throughout that weight-loss journey, she had experienced an internal emotional battle. She had identified that she had an inner conflict, but could not understand why she was still obsessed with food, even though she looked great and had achieved everything she wanted.

At the party, Ruth recalled that there was a buffet and she had found herself walking back and forth to it numerous times and stacking her plate high – basically binge-eating. Her weight had soon returned, and she was back to square one. She had felt great for losing the weight, but it had threatened her survival and caused the internal emotional pain to return, and so she had returned to binge-eating to silence the voice.

Ruth said a huge weight had been lifted off her shoulders after our day of therapy. She also said it was the first time she had actually acknowledged that the abuse she had suffered was over and that she did not need to fear being attacked any longer.

We kept in touch with Ruth for quite some years, and during that time she was astonished that getting to a healthy weight was no longer a battle. Bearing in mind that she had all her knowledge of diet and fitness at her disposal, it was just a matter of conditioning her schema, which was no longer required. She also went on to say that she did not want to be a UK size 10 or 12, she just wanted to feel comfortable in her clothes, and that meant being a size 14.

For the first time in her life, Ruth had obtained peace with her past and now had the healthy relationship she needed with food.

'I realised that I couldn't knowingly look to food for a way out when it had so clearly led me here. It wasn't hunger that beckoned me to eat more. It wasn't my stomach that needed to be reconciled. It was shame. It was guilt.'

Andie Mitchell[23]

CASE STUDY
Jo: Post-traumatic Stress Disorder

Early one morning, Jo was riding her scooter to work as she normally would, when suddenly a car pulled out in front of her. She hit the car and was catapulted into the air over the bonnet. Jo was left disabled and unable to work. Her memory and speech were affected, and she changed from being an incredibly vibrant, confident and outgoing woman to a shadow of her former self. She was now entirely reliant upon her partner, who became her full-time carer, was visited each day by a nurse and was diagnosed with post-traumatic stress disorder. Even more difficult to bear was the fact that, due to her accident, she had developed a phobia of travel, and as Jo was now living in the north of England and all her family were in the south, she was unable to visit them. She was devastated about this – a feeling which was magnified when her mum was diagnosed with cancer. Jo felt an enormous amount of guilt and sadness that she was unable to be there to support her mum; in fact, she thought she might never see her again.

Jo's life became very insular and she subsequently became depressed. Her PTSD and her anxiety about travel led her to start self-medicating with food to ease the physical and mental pain. She also felt a great deal of anger towards the driver of the car that had hit her, who seemed to show no remorse, either on the day or in the court hearings that followed.

Jo came to see us with regards to her PTSD because she desperately wanted to visit her mum, dad and family in the south of England. It was clear from her questionnaire that despite the accident having happened a few years earlier, she was still very much a victim of it. She was having flashbacks about what happened, and held a lot of resentment and anger. Although we could not help Jo with her disability, we did feel that if she were to get over her PTSD, that would not only resolve her phobia of travel, but also her need to self-medicate with food, which would likely make her more mobile.

We spoke with Jo about the events of that day and helped her to see things from a different perspective. We asked questions such as: had the driver's intention that day been to find her and knock her off her scooter? Could the driver's reaction after the accident be due to shock and fear rather than indifference?

Our discussions helped Jo to change her view of herself from that of a victim to a survivor of a very unfortunate accident. We also helped her to understand that although we couldn't change what happened that day, there were still many things she was able to achieve.

Having ascertained that Jo's feelings about the accident had changed, we felt that her treatment for PTSD had been successful, and she left us looking much brighter. The following day we travelled with Jo and her partner by car to the south of England to surprise her mum and family. To be able to witness that and be part of a tearful and emotional reunion was incredibly rewarding.

Some two years later, while conducting a meet-and-greet

at one of our theatre shows, we were thrilled to see Jo sitting in the front row. She had lost a lot of weight and looked amazing. During the Q&A section, she raised her hand and said that she did not have a question but had something she would like to share. She told everyone how she had met with us, and how we had helped her with her travelling phobia and PTSD. She candidly told everyone how she had been unable to sleep soundly, care for herself, walk or travel. She said, 'I am here today not only to watch the Speakmans' show, but also because I wanted to say a big thank-you to them both for the way they transformed my life. I am now able to travel, and because I have gained control of my life, I have gained control of my eating and have lost 3 stone in weight [42lb/19kg].' She then went on to say, 'I was also told I would never be able to walk again, but I would now like to show Nik and Eva something.'

With that, Jo stood up and took a few small steps towards us. She could only manage to walk slowly, but she was walking, and in that moment, we both started to cry with emotion. The first day we met Jo, she was a broken woman, physically unhealthy and unable to walk. We never imagined that two years later, a much slimmer, more confident and more mobile version of her would be walking towards us. That moment was one of the most incredible of our career, and we will always hold it close to our hearts.

We have kept in touch with Jo, who periodically contacts us on social media with updates. Her life has completely transformed. She has moved to the south of England, has a new partner, is able to walk and is getting stronger all the time. More than anything, she is now a slim, happy, confident, vibrant young woman, just as she was before her accident.

Overcoming PTSD or Trauma

We know that with the right help, support and therapy, in time anyone can overcome PTSD or trauma. We hope our tips will also offer you some help. Please ask yourself the following:

1. Was it personal to you?

This is a significant element in our work when helping someone with PTSD, as often the feeling that what happened was in some way personal traps you indefinitely in the status of victim. It is therefore important to look for evidence as to why it was not personal. For example, in the case study above, when we helped Jo to realise that the car driver did not target her, nor were they specifically looking for her, she was able to release herself from that trauma.

Violence in a relationship may feel personal, but the fact is that your partner wasn't being aggressive towards you, they were being aggressive towards a partner – they will have been aggressive to partners before you and will be to partners after you, because they have aggression issues. This also applies to being bullied or abused. Bullies bully and abusers abuse – it gives them a sense of power, because within themselves they feel powerless or inadequate.

Accepting that your trauma was not personal to you negates the belief that you are a target, allowing you to accept that you are no longer at risk. Once the risk has been eradicated, the need to be on high alert is also no longer necessary.

2. Do you feel guilty?

Feelings of guilt occur because you either feel responsible for a traumatic event or you think you made a bad choice.

Or perhaps you do not understand why you survived when others did not.

Guilt is only a valid response if you directly and deliberately orchestrated a traumatic event. Knowing you did not means that you are not at fault. It is important to realise that, had you known in advance what was going to occur, you would never have been there or would have done things differently. But you did not know, so you could not have changed the event.

3. Do you feel anger?

Feeling anger towards a perpetrator negatively affects you, not them. There is a saying that to hate someone is like you drinking poison and expecting them to die. They will not feel the repercussions of your emotions. If you have suffered, work on not allowing yourself to suffer any longer.

To do this, consider altering your emotions towards the perpetrator from hate to pity. Pity the fact that anyone can be so mean, cruel, jealous or violent. To have learned these behaviours suggests that they have had a life filled with such things. And to sustain these behaviours, they must continue to be affected by their own negative emotions and painful traumas.

4. Do you have flashbacks?

Flashbacks will occur until you resolve your pain and make peace with it. Although you will never forget a traumatic event, you can reduce your negative emotional attachment to it by shifting your perspective of yourself from that of victim to victor.

You will usually see the flashback through your own eyes. Look at the memory and imagine yourself leaving your body, so that you can view the event as a third party. Observing it as a bystander should allow you to consider an alternative perspective of what happened. You may still feel sad about the event, but you should feel less emotional about it.

5. Do you feel blame?

As we saw with Jo, who blamed all motor vehicles for her accident, and Ruth, who blamed herself for her abuse, if you have PTSD or are suffering from trauma that stops you from doing things, consider what or who you may be blaming. What are you no longer able to do or experience as a result of your trauma? Question why that place, thing or person could be deemed responsible. Imagine if you were in a court of law in front of a jury – what actual evidence would you have to blame yourself, a place, a thing or an object? Invariably you will find that you are blaming the wrong thing and protecting yourself from something that poses no danger to you.

> *We all have the ability to leave things in the past once we have accepted that we should move on. That includes old friends, former partners, careers and traumas, too.*

Cutting Ties

Once you have cut ties with your past trauma and allowed yourself to heal, the need to self-medicate, protect or punish yourself with overeating will no longer be necessary or desired.

Look through your timeline now and your answers to the questionnaire. Are there any events listed there that left you feeling traumatised, in danger or fearful? If you would score the negative emotion you feel when considering that event a six or more out of ten, then work through the points above for each trauma.

Address one trauma at a time, scoring your discomfort before and after, applying the suggestions we have made to help you overcome your trauma.

Freedom from our past traumas tastes better than any food.

8

Body Confidence and Self-esteem

I can honestly say that if I hadn't attended a workshop with Nik and Eva Speakman, I would NEVER have lost 3 stone [42lb/19kg] and kept it off for over three years now. I have a new relationship with food and, not only that, I am healthier and so much happier. Big hugs and thanks, both.

W.B.

Self-esteem

Having low self-esteem can be a significant component to weight gain, self-medicating with food and an inability to maintain a healthy weight.

Take a look in a mirror right now. How would you describe the person looking back at you? Are you using negative, unkind or even insulting words and descriptions? If the answer is yes, then you are suffering from low self-esteem.

Self-esteem is accepting who you are and how you look and loving yourself for who you are, both inside and out. Once this self-acceptance exists then it becomes a motivator that can drive you to be the best you can physically, mentally and emotionally be. It can also give you the drive, determination and enthusiasm to achieve your goals, whether they are personal or professional, and certainly those that are in relation to your health, weight and well-being.

It is therefore key to your weight-loss success that you attain inner peace, self-love and appreciation, as it is this that will help you generate confidence and enthusiasm and give you the necessary permission to make yourself happy.

NBC News reported in 2017 that 85 per cent of people suffer with low self-esteem.[24] This is a staggering figure! Could this also be why so many people in the US also suffer with weight issues?

People with low self-esteem can feel unloved, unworthy, insecure, ashamed, pessimistic, unhappy, guilty and very often depressed. This is the reason why people all too often reach for a quick pick-me-up in the form of high-calorie, sugary foods. This then leads to negative feelings of unworthiness or that you do not deserve the time investment that goes into exercise and being healthy.

If this sounds familiar, we would like to share an important point with you: how you perceive yourself is largely based upon how other people have made you feel about yourself. Therefore, your weight issues could be the result of your self-esteem having been knocked by someone else.

Here are some case studies of people who have all gained weight because of self-sabotaging as a consequence of low self-esteem. This will give you an insight into why anyone who has low self-esteem might struggle with their weight. As we have previously stated, knowing other people's stories and understanding why they did what they did and how they subsequently changed is a great way to identify the changes you might need to make and how you might go about doing so.

CASE STUDY
Gary: Low Self-esteem

Gary's memory of his mum was quite vague. He had sadly lost her when he was just three years of age, and was left with his dad and three elder brothers. He did have one specific memory, however, of cuddling up on the sofa, watching children's television with her. He recalled with fondness drinking milk and eating biscuits in this moment.

Gary's dad was working full time to keep a roof over their heads after his mum passed away, and he soon met someone else and remarried – possibly, Gary felt, to provide a mother and carer for his four children. Sadly, however, Gary described his dad's new wife as a stereotypical wicked stepmother from a fairytale.

He remembers often feeling hungry because she would taunt him and his brothers with cakes and treats but would not allow them to have any. When their father returned home from work, she would behave like a doting mother, telling their father not to give them any more cakes or biscuits, as they had eaten enough already before he came home.

Gary had a clear and vivid memory from when he was perhaps eight or nine years of age of waking up in the night feeling incredibly hungry. He went downstairs to the kitchen and took some biscuits, but his stepmother woke and caught him eating them. He remembers her chastising him, twisting and nipping his skin, and telling him that he was disgusting and fat.

From then on, Gary's stepmother habitually spoke down to Gary. And despite trying to keep his defiance under the radar, it appeared to make him all the more noticeable to his stepmother, who would then pick on him. When his father wasn't there, she was incredibly cruel. Gary recalled numerous occasions when his stepmother told him that his mother hadn't really died, that she had left the family because she hated Gary, and that it was only when Gary arrived that his mother left. When Gary was 12 or 13, she told him that his mother had killed herself because she hated Gary. She repeatedly told Gary that he had caused his mother's depression and suicide, and that if he had not been born, his mother would still be alive.

Gary grew up feeling loathed and confused. Although his dad was a kind and quiet soul, Gary did not feel able to talk to him about his stepmother or his own mother – which in any event, was a rule that had been brought in by his new wife.

The moment Gary was old enough to work, he left school so he could earn enough money to get away and gain some control over his life. He described his first home as a crumby bedsit, but it was his home, where he felt safe and could control what and how much he could eat. He vowed he would never go hungry again.

Understandably, having had his food restricted, Gary now started to overeat. As he worked in a fast-food restaurant, he would often eat there. His breakfast, lunch and dinner would generally consist of burgers, fries, cakes and other high-calorie foods. In view of the fact that Gary had absolutely no confidence as a consequence of his stepmother's put-downs throughout his life, he kept himself to himself and did not venture into having relationships. He felt that he was fat, ugly and did not deserve love.

When Gary was 38, he attended a motivational talk that we conducted, after which he booked on to one of our full-day workshops. While attending this workshop, Gary volunteered for our confidence demonstration.

As he bravely came on stage, he gave everyone a summary of his life and explained that he had no sense of self-worth and hated himself. As Gary spoke bravely about the life he had endured, the majority of the room began to cry. He told us how he had never known how his mother had died, but that, when attending a family funeral in his late twenties, his aunt had explained that she had died from cancer. Apparently, she had had some ailments that she had ignored and by the time her illness was discovered, it was too late to save her.

Despite being given this information, Gary did not fully absorb the magnitude of what he had been told, as he had created schemas in his childhood based on the belief that his mum had left him because he wasn't good enough. The truth should have freed him from the burden he carried, but Gary continued to believe what his stepmother had said, which continued to make him feel bad.

We asked Gary whether his aunt had any reason to lie to him. Gary said no. We asked whether any of his memories of his mum consisted of her being unkind, cruel or dismissive towards him. Gary said it was quite the contrary; the memories and photos he had all displayed a loving mum who was very kind. We then asked Gary why he was choosing his stepmother over his actual mother. He looked hurt and confused and said, 'I would never choose my stepmother over my own mum.' We pointed out that believing what his stepmother had told him over his own loving memories and the love he could see in his mum's expressions in the photos was tantamount to him choosing his stepmother over his own mother. We saw an instant shift in Gary when he said, 'I have never looked at it that way before, you are right.'

We then asked Gary: 'Did your mum choose to leave you?' Gary said no. We then asked: 'Why do you think your mum had four children?'

Gary answered, 'Because she must have wanted us.' We pointed out that after she had had one child, if she didn't want anymore, she wouldn't have done, yet she went on to have another three, proving that she enjoyed being a mum.

We then carried out a demonstration of our Mirror Technique with Gary (which we will share with you later in this chapter), and for the first time since the age of three, he saw himself through his mother's eyes – the eyes of true and unconditional love. The room fell silent. It was an emotional and beautiful moment.

Gary's attitude and demeanour changed immediately. He looked taller, happier, younger, lighter, and as he left the stage to a heartwarming round of applause, we were thrilled that Gary had had the courage to raise his hand and join us onstage. He was worthy and deserving of love and happiness, and we were confident that our words and mirror treatment had helped him.

At the end of the day, Gary came to speak to us to tell us how differently he was feeling. He also shared that other happy memories from his childhood were coming back to him, including days out, some fun memories with his dad and brothers and times when his dad had told him that he was the apple of his mum's eye.

Gary asked us why he might have blocked these memories out before, and we explained that, because of the emotional damage his stepmother had caused, she had overshadowed the happy memories and even the positive things his dad had told him. He had heard the words, but he wasn't listening. We offered the following analogy: that if he believed he was financially broke, yet we told him he wasn't, so he should go out and buy whatever he wanted, he would probably think, 'Yes, that would be nice, but I've got no chance of doing that, as I don't have any money.' A strong belief takes stronger evidence to alter it.

We were thrilled to meet Gary once more, as well as his fiancée, 18 months later at another workshop. His transformation was incredible. He looked handsome, had lost a lot of weight and was now working for an IT company. He told us that after leaving the workshop, he had realised it was time to love himself. We asked Gary whether the transition had been difficult. It was encouraging to hear him say, 'It was an effortless process, and one that was exciting.'

CASE STUDY
Eva: Low Self-esteem

I wanted to share my story with you because, although I have never been obese, I did battle with weight issues when I was at school, for which I was bullied.

I was born into a Polish family where food and eating were always key to every celebration, every gathering and every time a guest would visit our home. Our tradition was, and still is, to share food and drink when visitors arrive.

At home I didn't want for anything in terms of material possessions, but even so, life was turbulent, as my dad liked to drink. To others, life may have looked idyllic, but I was embarrassed about the fact that my mum and dad would argue, and that when Dad was drunk, he'd blow up both physically and verbally. I didn't want anyone to know what happened behind closed doors, so I avoided having friends over, and when I occasionally did, I was petrified of whether Dad would come home from work drunk or sober. If the worst happened and he was drunk, I'd have to laugh it off as if I'd never seen him drunk before and couldn't believe it!

I was never 'popular' at school, and at junior school was incredibly quiet. I did, however, have a best friend, who I adored. I would often go to her house to play, and I loved the calm I found there. When she moved away and left my school, I was so sad and felt incredibly lonely.

I have never liked conflict – on the contrary, I crave peace and calmness – so in my early teens, because I would never stand up for myself or retaliate, I was seen as an easy target for the school bullies.

I had one good friend when I was at senior school, though sadly our friendship only lasted two years, as she found another circle of friends outside of school who probably thought I was too quiet and uncool to join their gang. Again, I felt abandoned and alone.

Throughout this time, I comfort ate at school and therefore became a little plump. I recall having a little round tummy which I tried to hide with my school sweater, but still I got called 'fat' and even 'pregnant'. This comment really affected me. As an innocent 14-year-old, I was devastated, and this false, hurtful comment became a great topic of gossip and spread through the school like wild fire. It became so bad that I no longer wanted to go to school, but I was terrified that this would label me promiscuous, so after enduring years of bullying in silence, I felt that I had to speak out. I told my mum and she was furious. She went straight to see my head teacher to insist that the issue of the untrue pregnancy rumour was resolved, which thankfully it was, although the bullying was not.

After school I went to college and met my first boyfriend, who was very sweet, although that relationship totally fell apart when he cheated on me. Once again I felt totally crushed. My self-esteem and confidence sank lower than ever, and this cemented the schema I had previously created at school that I was fat and ugly! It seemed to offer even more evidence that it must be true.

I then met my second boyfriend, who started off as charming, but slowly started to chip away at me verbally, which over time developed into extreme violence. I made excuses for the way he acted and rationalised it. I blamed the drink, his friends, and I justified how awful he was by telling myself that he really loved me, while ignoring the overwhelming evidence to the contrary.

> *We accept what we are willing to tolerate, we tolerate what we believe we deserve.*

Our relationship finally came to an end after I was hospitalised with a serious head injury and he had punched my dad in the face. I felt like I could tolerate and may even have deserved being hit, but my dad did not. Him hurting my dad gave me the strength to finally walk away from him. My self-esteem was on the floor and I did not have the emotional skills to work through how I felt about myself, so I would silence my self-loathing with food and then over-exercise to try to compensate.

And then I met Nik . . .

Nik was like no one I had ever met before. He came from a sedate, loving, supportive family. He was calm, positive and sensible. He could turn everything into something positive and bombarded me with kindness and compliments – and at that time, this was not my type. The nicer he was, the more I pushed him away.

Looking back, I now realise I was self-sabotaging, as my expectation was that he would break my heart or cheat on me, because that was what had happened before.

However, Nik did not give up on me. He insisted on taking me to courses, training days, motivational talks and goal-setting workshops. We would listen to self-improvement tapes, and he would read me relevant parts of the many books he had previously read.

Thanks to Nik, I decided to accept responsibility for everything that had happened to me. I realised that there would only be one person with me 24 hours a day, seven days a week, for the rest of my life, and that person was me, and I deserved better.

As soon as I realised this and took action, I started to move on and change the patterns that were marring my life. My attitude to myself entirely changed. I was excited to become fit and healthy. I started to enjoy exercise and doing things for myself. I did not feel controlled by food, nor did I feel the need to self-medicate with it, as my ailment – my self-loathing – had been fixed.

Now I eat well, but also allow myself to have junk food on occasion, because I know I am in control. In the past, I could never understand how someone could have one biscuit, one small piece of cake or a handful of nuts or crisps without devouring the lot. I am delighted to share that this is possible for someone who has issues with food – I am living proof of it. To help you further, we will share our healthy-eating plan, our way of eating and our delicious but healthy recipes later in the book.

Raising Your Self-esteem

It is common to overlook your own qualities and attributes and see yourself through a lens of negativity imposed by others, without ever questioning their motive. But when you change the way you look at circumstances, the circumstances themselves can begin to change. It is therefore essential to build up your self-esteem.

You should first consider whether you might have misread a situation that has affected your self-esteem. For example, you may have overheard a conversation and thought someone was speaking negatively about you, when they were actually talking about someone else.

If you are certain that is not the case, however, here are some tips to build your self-esteem, which in turn will help to increase your confidence:

* Write a list of all the people who have made you feel bad. Were they a school bully, parent, teacher, colleague, partner, ex-partner?

* Now look at the list and consider whether this person (or people) is still a part of your life. If not, this suggests that you or they have moved on. Either way, they are in the past. Just as you have moved on with your life, you now need to decide to move on with your emotions, too.

* If they are still in your life, consider whether you can distance yourself from them. If not, tell them how they make you feel – you could write them a letter or speak to them in private.

* If you can't change them, you must change how you deal with them. For example, if they are very negative towards you, try being excessively positive in return. If they criticise you, say something like, 'That was hurtful, but I'll assume you're having a bad day, as I know you're too nice to be intentionally mean.' A different approach will provide a different result.

* Look at the list again, and ask yourself what skills, qualities or qualifications each person has (or had) to judge you. Why would you choose to allow their views to tarnish your view of yourself?

* Consider what their motive might have been to say or do such hurtful things to you.

* Next, ask yourself why you would want to carry unkind opinions around with you. If you are speaking to yourself negatively using their words, or as a consequence of

their actions, you are reinforcing their original unkind behaviour and picking up where they left off. If you see yourself as a kind person, remember that this should include being kind to yourself.

* Think again about the motives of the people who judged you. It is important to accept that you may have been their victim then, but today you are a survivor of those situations.

* Realise that if you have ever been loved, this is because you are lovable. Whether the person who loved you was a parent, sibling, friend or even a pet, consider the reasons why they love or loved you.

What a difference a year makes. I'm now 1.5 stone [21lb/9.5kg] lighter. Thank you for helping me start my weight-loss journey.

Katie

The Mirror Technique

Seeing Yourself Through the Eyes of Love

Now that you have dealt with the people in your life who have unjustifiably made you feel bad about yourself, we would like to share with you a technique that we often use, which helps to increase self-worth, self-esteem and self-love. We want you to gift yourself the health and happiness you deserve. You will need a notepad and pen, a voice recorder on your telephone or a trusted friend to make notes for you.

Stand in front of a full-length mirror. While looking in the mirror, write down or record everything that you see and say about yourself. What kind of person do you see in front of you? Are they weak? Are they strong? What do you look like? Do you see any weaknesses? If so, what are they? Write everything you perceive about yourself. Describe the person in front of you, both visually and emotionally. How do you feel about that person? Look at all your body parts and write down what you see.

Once you have written the list, count how many of the things you have said about yourself are negative and how many are positive.

We would now like you to write a list of just the negative things that you have said about yourself. Look at those words and ask yourself, 'Would I ever say those negative things to a stranger?' If not, why not? Would you ever say them to a friend? If not, why not?

Again, looking at the negative things you have said about yourself, consider whether you would ever say them to your child, partner, parents or loved ones. If not, why not?

Now consider that if you would never say the things you said about yourself to someone you love or to a friend, family member or even to a stranger, that must be because those words are mean and unkind. And if it is not acceptable to say those things to anybody else, it is absolutely not acceptable to say those things to yourself.

Now we would like you to look at those negative things you have said about yourself and consider who has said these things to you or made you feel this way. Use the list from the exercise above, or write a new list of anybody you feel has contributed to these negative, unkind comments, then look at that list and ask:

* **Why would you want to listen to that person?**

* **What qualifications do they have to judge you?**

* Are they even a part of your life? If not, that is because they are not important to you. However, if they are still a part of your life, then consider why they may have said those things to you.

* Is it because they were envious or jealous of you?

* Is it because you have or had something they wanted (e.g. a nice family, a nice home, skills or qualities they envied, etc.)?

* Is it because they were scared of losing you? Perhaps by knocking your self-esteem, they thought you were less likely to leave them and find a new friend/partner and likely to appreciate them more.

* Is it because that person felt bad about themselves and in an effort to make themselves feel better they had to knock you down?

* Is it because they feared you would steal their limelight? Maybe in front of a friend, parent, teacher, or a boy or girl they were attracted to?

* Is it because they were worried that you might supersede them in life?

Once you have considered these things and realised that the words you used to describe yourself aren't yours but based upon somebody else's or how somebody else has made you feel, it's time to move on to the next part of the Mirror Technique, in which we would like you to view yourself through the eyes of love to see your true inner beauty.

If you have a voice recorder on your phone or a tape recorder that would be most effective, as this exercise is far more beneficial if you can keep your eyes closed. If not, keep your eyes closed, and then write down everything positive that you can remember once you have actually completed the next part of the technique.

Stand in front of the mirror and close your eyes. If you are a little bit unsteady, you may want to put a chair beside you to give you something to hold on to. Alternatively, you can sit on the chair if you are unable to stand.

With your eyes closed we would like you to think of someone who loves you unconditionally, either now or in the past. That may be a partner, a parent, a best friend, a colleague, a teacher, a pet or even someone who has passed away, like a grandparent. Just think of somebody who has or does love you unconditionally.

Still with your eyes closed, imagine that person standing beside you, shoulder to shoulder. Now imagine that you are floating out of your body and into that person's body, and looking through their eyes at your reflection in the mirror.

What we would now like you to do – and hopefully you can record this – is to say out loud all the things that person sees or saw in you. So, looking through your loved one's eyes at your reflection in the mirror, say out loud what that person loves about you. What do they see? How do they describe you? Why do they love you?

For example:

* **Do they tell you that they love you?**

* **Do they say you are beautiful, kind, intelligent, fun to be around, that you are loyal, perfect, a good cook, a good housekeeper, good at doing something in particular or good at making them feel special or loved?**

* **What do they say about your looks? Do they compliment you about your hair, eyes, figure, stature or smile?**

Now, in the knowledge that the person who loves or loved your is not a liar and that their feelings towards you were honest and true, say out loud all the compliments that person has ever given you and everything they love and feel about you. Say it as they said it, repeating their words four or five times with all the love, sincerity and meaning they were gifting to you.

Alternatively, use your recording. Press play, and with your eyes closed again, imagine seeing yourself in the mirror through the eyes of your loved one and listen to all the words that person said about you, everything they love about you. Listen to the words four or five times.

If you can't do this with a voice recording, that is absolutely fine. Using the exact same process, just try to remember the person's words instead, and then say them out loud four or five times over.

Once you have done this, very slowly open your eyes and see yourself in that mirror for the first time through the eyes of love. See yourself in the knowledge that the person who said all those lovely things about you did so because they were true, because people do not give compliments without reason. Nor do people give love without reason. Love is earned, and if anyone has ever loved you unconditionally, that is because *you* have earned it and because you are lovable.

Now write down all those compliments and positive things that your loved one said about you and keep them somewhere prominent. This could be at the side of your bed, on the sun-visor in your car, in your desk at work, in your bag or wallet, on the refrigerator door or in all of these places. Whenever you need to remind yourself of how amazing you are, how loved you are and that you deserve to be happy, healthy and to have a positive relationship with food, reread this list and hear your loved one's voice as you do so.

Finally, return to your timeline, look at your list of positive events and then consider any happy occasions you may have forgotten to add, such as a time when you laughed uncontrollably, when you fell in love (either with a person, place or pet), when you were given a compliment or achieved something, or a special place or memorable experience. Now you can invest in yourself by often remembering how incredible you are and what fabulous things you have seen, experienced, tried and been part of.

9

Junk-food Addiction

I haven't eaten chocolate since [your workshop] and don't want to either . . . I had the best day – thank you again.

Sally

Many people, including those whose stories we have shared in this book, who have had issues with excess weight, a poor diet and overeating, use the words 'junk-food addict' to describe themselves. But whether we are speaking to someone who believes they are addicted to drugs, smoking, coffee, alcohol or food, our response – though perhaps controversial to some or blatantly obvious to others – is always the same: '*We do not believe that the addiction is the problem. We believe the cause is the issue.*'

If you are feeling unfulfilled in your life, if you are carrying around pain from your past, if you are stressed at work, if you have a problem, if you have a void in your life, if you need love or want a treat to celebrate, like most people, you may turn to food – usually junk food.

The reason people turn to junk food is that sweet or processed foods have a significant effect on the reward area of the brain. Feel-good neurotransmitters such as dopamine can be rapidly released by these unhealthy foods, therefore food addiction is not caused by greediness or a lack of willpower; it is due to the fact that, for some reason, you feel a need for the feel-good effects the junk food provides.

If you find that you are craving unhealthy foods even though you are not hungry, or that you cannot resist the urge to eat high-calorie, high-sugar and high-fat foods, then you could be considered a 'junk-food addict'.

No chocolate, crisps or cake for a week. It's amazing.

D. Andrea

Symptoms of Junk-food 'Addiction'

1 When you start eating junk food, you feel you can't stop.

2 You crave junk food, even if you feel full.

3 When you give in and start eating a food you craved, you often find yourself eating much more than you intended.

4 If you make a decision not to eat junk food, you find yourself obsessing about it and not being able to push it out of your mind.

5 You feel guilty after eating a large quantity of junk food, yet you return to it the moment you can.

6 You have tried, but you feel powerless to stop eating junk food.

7 You feel ashamed about eating junk food, so sometimes eat it in secret.

8 You make excuses to justify why you should allow yourself to eat junk food. For example, you say that you feel stressed, you have had a challenging day, you need the energy or that you have eaten very little that day.

9 Your diets and healthy-eating intentions are sabotaged and fail as a result of giving in to the urge to eat junk food.

10 You feel angry, defensive or sad if anyone tries to stop you from eating junk food when you want to eat it.

Facts and Causes

Junk food triggers the pleasure centres of the brain and releases feel-good chemicals such as dopamine and serotonin. Common causes of junk-food addiction can include:

Past unresolved emotional issues

Eating junk food may be a form of self-medicating unresolved issues from your past that have gone on to cause negative feelings and emotions such as sadness, confusion, guilt and low self-esteem.

Reward

You may use junk food to rekindle the comfort and positive emotions of your childhood, when foods such as chocolate and sweets were given as a reward, treat or celebration, therefore creating positive associations with those foods.

Tiredness, exhaustion and insomnia

You may feel you need sugars and simple carbohydrates to provide a quick boost of energy and to satisfy hunger caused by the increased release of ghrelin (the hormone that creates the feeling of hunger) when tired or sleep-deprived.

Depression

When feeling low, junk food can be a go-to – an accessible form of temporary self-medication. It can help both to distract and, due to the benefits of the dopamine and serotonin that it releases, temporarily elevate your mood.

Low self-esteem

In addition to temporarily elevating mood, junk food can also be a tool used to sabotage or punish yourself by gaining weight to feel less attractive or confident – a consequence of when you have been made to feel inadequate in the past.

Copying

We are a product of our environment. Just as we copy our accent from our parents, we will also often copy their eating patterns, including their portion sizing as our reference for what is acceptable.

Heartache or loneliness

Eating can help to offer a distraction when lonely or healing a broken heart. The brief elevated mood can offer some short-term comfort.

Substance abuse

Junk food can satisfy the urge to eat created by alcohol, drugs or the come down from both.

Void filler

Eating can often help to fill a void and offers a distraction when lonely or bored or if we have too much time on our hands.

Stress, anxiety or upset

For those unsure how to deal with daily issues, problems, upsets and anxieties, junk food can offer a quick, easy and accessible source of temporary relief or distraction.

I attended [your workshop] last September – since then I've changed so much. Haven't eaten crisps or chocolate since. I've lost 2.5 stone [35lb/16kg].

Sophia

CASE STUDY
Rick: Junk-food Addiction

Rick told us that he had an addiction to junk food that stopped him from achieving the physique he knew he could and should have. He said that once he started eating any form of junk food, particularly fast food, he didn't just eat it – he devoured it. Often, he would not even taste or appreciate the food, because he would just 'shovel it down his throat'.

From his timeline and questionnaire, we learned that Rick was an only child and would often be rewarded with treats and fast food by his mum after school. After some discussion it became evident that as a result of this, he had created a schema that fast food and junk food equalled reward, appreciation and love.

Later in life, Rick took a great interest in his health and physique and attended the gym regularly. He looked good, yet on occasion he would binge-eat junk food, and this was something he wanted our help with, as it was sabotaging his weight goals and his dream of competing in a bodybuilding competition.

He was angry and disappointed with himself when he binged, which would then give him an excuse to repeat his binge, after which he would feel even more disgusted at the volume of food he had managed to consume in one go.

Our therapy is evidential, and so to help us unravel and address Rick's issue and identify any patterns to his behaviour, we asked him to complete a food diary over a two-week period before meeting with us. From looking at the diary, we could see an obvious acceleration in his consumption of unhealthy junk foods on certain days. When we asked him to tell us what had occurred on those days, he was embarrassed to admit that the bingeing was common if he ever drank alcohol to excess or took drugs.

As a result of all the information we had obtained from his food diary, timeline and questionnaire, we identified a schema that needed to be addressed, which was that '*junk food provides love and reward*'. We would tackle the drinking and drug-taking later, but first we asked Rick to tell us about when he was taken to fast-food restaurants as a child. He confirmed that his mum would pick him up and take him straight from school. We then asked if he would later sit down with his parents for dinner. Rick thought about that for a few moments, and then told us that, as he had already eaten, he would not have dinner with his parents. In any event, his father, who had his own business, would work very late, so he would rarely see him on weekday evenings.

As a result of this discussion, Rick then had a huge realisation. Looking back, he could not recall his mum cooking dinner often. We asked Rick: 'Are you saying that your mum would take you to a fast-food restaurant because she didn't want to cook dinner?'

Rick was amused that he had not identified this before, and said, 'I can see that this is probably what happened

– my mum hated cooking.' He then went on to tell us that they would sometimes joke about his mum's inability to cook anything beyond beans or cheese on toast. They would usually only sit down together as a family for dinner at the weekends, and even then, this would be at a local restaurant or pub. Rick was blown away that he had never realised this before. He had thought he was being taken for a treat after school, but in fact, his mum was taking him there to save her having to cook his dinner. We asked Rick to repeat to us why he had been taken out for burgers and fried chicken after school, so that he could absorb the truth, as opposed to his inaccurate childhood impression.

We then went on to carry out our Bungee Technique to alter Rick's perspective on fast food and chocolate (which we will share later in this chapter, see page 167). We helped to make these foods less appealing by strongly associating them with olives, which he hated so much they would make him gag. Once we were confident that Rick's former inaccurate schema had been updated and conditioned, we moved on to discuss his use of alcohol and drugs.

We explained to Rick that, while we are chemically impaired, we are unable to override the effects of drugs and alcohol, which studies suggest influence the hormones associated with hunger and identifying when we are full. Furthermore, when under the influence of alcohol, cognition, behaviour and choices are often affected. We were particularly interested, however, in why Rick felt he needed to drink and take drugs in the first place. Was this a form of self-medication? Was this an addiction? Was it even self-harm? Or did he perceive this as fun and relaxation? We wanted to understand Rick's positive intent, which he would undoubtedly use to justify his use of drugs and excess alcohol, to see if this was also an area we could positively impact.

It transpired that Rick's drug and alcohol use was primarily orientated around a particular group of friends. This was their habit and he would give in to peer pressure and follow suit, because he liked these friends and wanted to belong to their group.

As Rick was an only child, we understood his desire to belong, but we explained that, although we had addressed his schema associated with junk food, no amount of therapy could override the effects drugs and alcohol have on hunger, fullness and choices made whilst under the influence. As a grown man, he now had a decision to make: he could choose to indulge in drink and drugs with those friends, he could abstain from seeing the friends or he could choose not to drink or take drugs when he was with them.

When we next saw Rick he told us his relationship with junk food had improved. His desire for it had diminished since realising that he had previously seen it as a reward but had got it wrong. Our session had taught him that junk food was not a reward; on the contrary, for him, it was more like a punishment, as it impeded his goals of achieving a great physique. This realisation had significantly altered his perception of junk food and subsequently his relationship with it. He now consciously chose better rewards for himself, such as watching his favourite TV show or a movie, having a sports massage or taking his new partner out. Indeed, Rick went on to explain that his issue with regards to his friends had also largely resolved itself, because now that he was dating someone new, he did not see them so often or for long periods.

Six days after attending the Speakmans' event and I have not had or desired a bar of chocolate. It is incredible!

Jill

How to Help Your Junk-food Addiction

1 Look at resolving the issues that cause you to crave the release of feel-good hormones through junk food to feel better. Do this with the help of your questionnaire and timeline.

2 Look at your food diary to identify when you overindulge and if you are with someone when it happens.

3 Consider saboteurs to your success, such as lack of sleep, people you associate with, alcohol or drugs.

4 List the foods that encourage your junk-food addiction, such as chocolate, chips, burgers, etc.

5 Go through your list of foods from step 4 and either find a healthier alternative for each or carry out our Bungee Technique (see page 167) to help make these foods unappealing.

Hi Nik and Eva. No chocolate since your workshop.
Half a stone less [7lb/3kg]. Half-marathon back to 1 hour
40 minutes after many years! Thank you!

David

Changing your perspective on the food you know you shouldn't eat

Many years ago, we perfected a simple technique to help change peoples' perspective on the foods that sabotage their weight-loss success. We started to demonstrate this technique, which we refer to as our Bungee Technique, at our workshops and the results were overwhelming. We were delighted to learn that people were able to watch our demonstration and then successfully apply the technique themselves at home.

The Bungee Technique is based on linking the foods you love to foods you would never eat – preferably foods that make you wretch or feel nauseous at the very thought of them. In the science world, this is referred to as conditioned taste aversion (CTA).

CTA, also known as the Garcia Effect, was first observed in the work of American psychologist Dr John Garcia in the 1950s. Dr Garcia conducted experiments with rats and discovered that, having given them water sweetened with saccharin and a chemical to make them sick, the rats associated the sweetened water with being sick. Once the association had been made, the rats would not drink or taste the sweetened water anymore, despite being hungry and thirsty. Dr Garcia had found that taste aversion is an acquired reaction to the smell or taste that an animal is exposed to before getting sick.[25]

This would explain why our method is so effective – particularly when carried out using a food that really makes you feel sick or nauseous.

Personally, we have not eaten crisps or chocolate for over 12 years now, having practised the technique on ourselves. The best thing of all about the method is that, if carried out correctly, the desire to eat these foods is extinguished indefinitely.

Hey, you two lovely people! Hope you're both okay. So, everything is still going well with the weight loss, still on the right track and I've lost more since the weigh-in. I haven't touched chocolate, which for me is incredible!

*And I cannot thank you enough for that, it was my biggest
downfall. I still think of tuna, which puts me off, then I think
of why I wanted to avoid chocolate in the first place. I'm
really enjoying my new healthier lifestyle, and I'm seeing
the results, especially in my clothes.*

Vicky

The Bungee Technique

Our Bungee Technique is designed to make some of those
sweet temptations far less appealing. First, look at your food
diary and notice which foods are your vice foods – the ones
that sabotage your weight loss. The most common ones are
chocolate, sweets, cake or crisps.

We discovered that everybody has individual coding.
What we mean by this is that we all see things in a
certain, often unique, way. To demonstrate this, we would
now like you to imagine the face of somebody you love
unconditionally, someone who is a big part of your life. That
might be your partner, parent, child or pet. Now, imagine
where you feel a picture of their face would be in front of
yours (you may prefer to do this with your eyes closed). Just
imagine seeing their face and put your hand where you can
see it. Most people will notice that it feels as if the picture
is in front of them, very close to their face, maybe slightly
to the left or right. Put your hand where you see or feel the
image of their face, and notice its particular position.

Try this again but thinking about another person you
really care about. Close your eyes if you prefer, imagine their
face and again put your hand where you can see or feel it.
Again, you will notice that it feels as though their picture is
close to you.

Now try this with a person you haven't seen for a long
time, somebody who isn't that important to you – maybe

somebody you went to school with or even an old teacher. This time, you should notice that the person's image feels further away and perhaps not as clear.

Having carried out this exercise, you will notice that you code important people in your life as close to you, whereas those who are less important are further away.

You code foods in a similar way; we have identified that people's vice foods, which they absolutely love, are always incredibly close to them, and those that they would never eat are incredibly far away.

If you would now like to change your perspective on the foods that sabotage your healthy-eating plans, consider a food that you would rather no longer desire (you will have to do this with one food at a time). We will use chocolate as an example while explaining our technique.

Just as you did with the people you cared about, close your eyes and imagine where you see the chocolate. If chocolate is something you love, you will notice that the image of chocolate feels quite close to you. It is also very likely that it will be clear and brightly coloured. Notice what you see, and where you see it, then physically put your hand where you can see it and open your eyes. Remember where you positioned the chocolate, and then put your hand down.

Now think of something you would never eat. Something that makes you feel nauseous, has previously made you vomit or that you just could never or would never try. It is best to use a food product. Some examples that people have used when we have conducted this exercise have included tripe, raw liver, raw fish, squid, sour milk and offal. However, be sure to choose your own food, as it may be something that other people would enjoy, such as olives or tuna fish. Whatever it is, it must be something that you would never eat.

Once you have chosen the food, close your eyes and imagine where you code this food. For this example, we will use tripe. You will probably notice that the food you wouldn't want to eat is coded quite far away. Most people will see it not only further away, but also very low down, close to or on the floor, but this will be personal to you. Be aware of where you see this food and then open your eyes and notice where it would be. Is it at the other end of the room? Outside the window? Was the image clear or unclear?

The next part of this technique is to move the food you enjoy to the position of the food that you would never eat. You can do this with your eyes open or you can close them if that is easier for you. Imagine that the food you like – in this example, chocolate – which is likely close up, is on a tight bungee cord. Then imagine yourself cutting the cord and releasing the chocolate, and watching it fly to and land in the food you would never eat – in our example, tripe. Do this four or five times: see yourself releasing the chocolate and allowing it to drop right onto the tripe and become tangled in the stomach-churning stuff.

Each time you allow the chocolate to fall into the tripe, close your eyes and see the chocolate in the distance mixing with the tripe, with the juices from the tripe running through the chocolate. Start to diminish the colour and clarity of this image to replicate how you saw the tripe. Imagine how the chocolate looks now, grey and wet and tainted by the tripe, and the smell of the tripe and chocolate combined, before slowly opening your eyes.

Repeat this exercise until you feel the same queasiness about the chocolate that you did when thinking about the tripe. You should now notice that when you think of chocolate, it is far in the distance with the tripe. If this is the case, then the technique is complete. If not, and the chocolate is still close or closer than the tripe, you will need to repeat this exercise until they become inextricably intertwined.

Once this technique has been successfully carried out, you may find that, subject to your personal coding, you do not desire any chocolate at all, or, if you have individually recoded different chocolate bars, you may need to repeat the Bungee Technique with different varieties. Most people, however, find that chocolate has been recoded as one group, and therefore they do not need to repeat this with individual chocolate types. However, you should not test this by eating some, as you could recode chocolate back to where it was. Also, beware when drinking alcohol, as this could lead you to doing things you would not normally wish to, and could result in you trying chocolate, enjoying it and creating a new positive coding towards it.

Lovely to meet you. I did your chocolate exercise with meat. Could not eat it the next day.

M.K.

Well, you guys started my weight-loss programme when I came to your seminar in Birmingham three or four years ago now . . . I still think of liver when I see a packet of crisps . . . thank you so much, I'm now 3 stone lighter and three dress sizes smaller . . . and I've kept it off . . . yes, you are angels x

Wendy

10

Yo-yo Dieting

The average weight gain for dieters will actually be greater than those who never diet. This happens because non-dieters learn that the food supply is reliable so there is less need for the insurance of fat stores.

Dr Andrew Higginson,
Senior Psychology Lecturer, University of Exeter[26]

Yo-yo dieting or weight cycling is a pattern of behaviour where you lose weight and then gain it again, and therefore your weight fluctuates up and down like a yo-yo.

Yo-yo dieting is very common, and you will find that many of the reasons why you lose and then gain weight are similar to those shared in Chapter 9 (see page 159). However, there are other factors that might affect why you find yourself going on a diet with enthusiasm, noticing that you feel and look better, and then slowly but surely falling back into your old bad habits. In our opinion, this pattern of behaviour is a symptom, the most probable cause of which is going on a diet in the first place.

Only those who diet can be affected by yo-yo dieting.

Why Diets Don't Work

We are huge fans of healthy eating and promoting a healthy mind, a healthy environment, movement and hydration. We are not, however, fans of diets, and in this chapter we will explain why.

As we see it, diets do not work long term. They are a great tool for short-term goals, such as losing weight for a wedding or holiday, but they are rarely sustainable over a long period of time. The reasons for this are that most diets do not incorporate the foods you most enjoy, nor do they address how much you eat, what you eat, when you eat, why you eat what you do and why you have the desire to eat when you are not hungry.

> *Restriction leads to desire.*

In one way or another, diets mean restriction. When you tell yourself that you cannot have something you want, the consequence is quite often an obsession with that food. After all, a restrictive diet plan is someone else's plan for you. Often, after you eat what you are told to eat for your breakfast, you will then be preoccupied with the diet's expectations of you for lunch, and after lunch you think about what you have to prepare for dinner. The following day, the cycle resumes.

The simple fact is that diets rarely work. According to Traci Mann, a professor of psychology at UCLA and lead author of a rigorous analysis of diet studies, 'Diets do not lead to sustained weight loss or health benefits for the majority of people.'[27]

Yes, you may lose weight, but does that weight loss last? Often it does not, and you fall into a cycle of yo-yo dieting. As each diet fails, you will likely feel bad and disappointed in yourself. You may feel guilty or, even worse, like a failure, and these emotions will ultimately knock your self-esteem even more. You will naturally blame yourself, as opposed to the impracticality of the diet plan, or the lack of emotional support or evaluation that it provides, as the reason for your weight gain.

Diets can also be counterproductive. Quick-fix extreme diets are guaranteed to launch you into yo-yo dieting, as they are often not sustainable or even healthy in the long term. Diets orientated around shakes, pills and bars can lead to you feeling isolated or appearing antisocial as you are unable to join family and friends for dinners and celebrations. And although most diets will help you to lose weight, as you lose fat during periods of intense dieting, your levels of the hormone leptin – which helps you to feel full – also reduce. This can lead to an increased appetite as the body tries to resupply its depleted energy stores. It is therefore far more beneficial to opt for a life of healthy eating, as opposed to dieting, in order to give your body a steady supply of energy and healthy fuel, while sensibly losing weight and creating a new, more positive way of eating.

> With studies of the long-term outcomes showing that at least one-third of dieters regain more weight than they lost, together with prospective studies indicating that dieting during childhood and adolescence predicts future weight gain and obesity, there is concern as to whether dieting may paradoxically be promoting exactly the opposite of what it is intended to achieve.
>
> Department of Medicine, Psychology Division, University of Fribourg, Switzerland[28]

New research carried out by Exeter and Bristol universities has suggested that repeated dieting leads to weight gain because the brain interprets the diet as a short-term famine, therefore encouraging the person to store more fat for future shortages.[29] This is likely to be a significant cause of why many people who fail on a diet then go on to gain more weight and become heavier than they were before they started the diet. In contrast, the studies also found that people who do not diet allow their body to learn that food supplies are constant and reliable, and therefore they do not need to store excess fat.

> *Diets convince your brain to store fat, whereas more fat stores cause you to diet.*

This is a vicious circle. Every diet you embark upon convinces your brain that famines are likely, and in a bid to protect you, your body will gain and hold weight until your brain has been retrained to trust that a steady supply of food and nutrients is available, which can take some time.

Healthy-eating Saboteurs

Tiredness

Sleep-deprivation is a risk factor for weight gain, as it affects the levels of two hormones that control our feelings of hunger and fullness (ghrelin and leptin).

A lack of sleep raises production of ghrelin, which is an appetite stimulant. This would explain why you may find that you eat more in the evening or when you are feeling tired.

Leptin, on the other hand, tells your brain when you are full, and a lack of sleep reduces its production, so you will eat more before feeling satisfied.

Feeling tired will also stand in the way of exercise, as it diminishes your enthusiasm to make the effort. And finally, if you are not sleeping enough, your body will release more insulin after eating, which promotes fat storage.[30] Obtaining enough sleep is therefore essential to your weight-loss success.

Alcohol

You may have noticed that your appetite and food consumption increases during and after drinking alcohol. The effects of alcohol undoubtedly lower your willpower and interfere with your clarity of thought and good intentions.

> **Alcohol switches the brain into starvation mode, increasing hunger and appetite, scientists have discovered.**[31]
>
> **Michelle Roberts,**
> **health editor, BBC News online**

Tests on mice have also highlighted, however, that alcohol activated their brain signals, which told them to eat more food. The alcohol caused increased activity in the neurons that are present when the body experiences starvation, which in turn creates intense hunger. It is believed that the effects of alcohol on the human brain are the same, which would explain why overeating is linked with its consumption. We would therefore urge you to consider the frequency of your alcohol consumption, as neither we, our therapy nor any healthy-eating plan can counteract the effects of alcohol. It is also high in calories, so avoiding it will help you to maintain a healthier weight.

People should be made aware of the impact alcohol
can have on how much they eat and what they eat,
along with the associated health risks.

Michelle Roberts,
health editor, BBC News online[32]

Drugs and medication

Taking drugs such as marijuana will impair your perception,
your concentration, your cognition and your ability to learn,
problem solve, make decisions or focus on given tasks. Long-
term use of drugs such as cocaine can also permanently alter
the reward area of the brain, making the user less sensitive to
dopamine.[33] In consequence, the user needs to take stronger,
larger and more frequent quantities of drugs to create
the same high, or may seek more stimulants to reach this
unnatural level of euphoria.

Many people we have helped have told to us that,
although cocaine can be an appetite suppressant, it is often
the case that the moment the effects start to wear off,
users go on to binge-eat, usually desiring unhealthy high-
sugar, high-fat foods. The withdrawal symptoms from some
drugs can include depression, low mood, fatigue, insomnia,
impaired concentration and increased appetite – all of which
can promote unhealthy eating and an increased desire to
eat to elevate your mood. We would strongly recommend
avoiding recreational drugs at all costs.

To ensure that all possibilities are addressed in your
weight-loss journey, it is also worth researching the potential
side effects of any medications that you take, as many
prescription medicines can increase your appetite or cause
weight gain. Some examples could be corticosteroids,
antidepressants, diabetes medications, contraceptives or
hormone-related medications. It is also a good idea to speak
with your doctor if you suspect that your medication is

affecting your weight and eating patterns, so that you can explore more favourable alternatives that might be available.

Hormones

Hormonal imbalances can create changes in our metabolism, causing a desire to overeat. If you feel that this is relevant to you, we would urge you to speak with your doctor, who will be able to offer tests, guidance or a referral to an endocrinologist if necessary.

Be assured, however, that even with a hormonal imbalance, you can still make positive changes to your lifestyle that will boost your self-confidence and encourage you to move more, look for opportunities to laugh and adopt a healthier approach to eating.

For example, another contributor to fat storage around the abdominal area can be anxiety, as a result of elevated levels of the stress hormone cortisol, so it is important to take action to reduce stress and anxiety in your daily life. Our book *Conquering Anxiety* could help you to identify and address your past stresses using your timeline and questionnaire, as well as actively alleviate your daily stresses. Effective time planning, delegating, talking, learning to say no, asking for help when needed, exercising, doing yoga, laughing, maintaining a good diet, taking up fun hobbies, hugging, spending time with good friends (while avoiding negative ones) and getting good-quality sleep can all be very helpful in reducing stress.

Unclear or unachievable goals

Would you ever consider getting into a car or onto a train if you had no idea where you were going? Imagine if you knew you desperately needed to be somewhere but had no idea of the address. You would feel incredibly frustrated, and no matter how hard you tried, no matter how good your intentions or how focused and motivated you might be, you would inevitably fail in your mission.

This is one of the most significant contributors to people's weight-loss failures. It is not enough to say, 'I am going to lose weight.' If you want to lose weight, be healthy and maintain your motivation, you need to have a clear, defined, written goal. If your goal is just to lose weight, then as soon as you have lost your first pound, you will have succeeded, and you will lose your motivation. Once you have a specific weight or dress size to aim for, your motivation will come from achievement, and if you are able to see that you are taking small steps in the right direction, this will help to keep you on track. If you know where you are now and where you want to be, and are able to identify the progress you have made each week, you will be much more likely to succeed in losing weight.

Your goals should always be realistic, broken down into manageable steps, to allow you to celebrate and appreciate your achievements along the way. For example, if you aim to lose half a pound per week, you are more likely to achieve this and more besides, meaning you will not only see your goal achieved, but also, if you have lost more, feel extra proud of your efforts, which will help to keep you motivated.

Another goal you could set yourself is to be more active. This could start with a simple goal of walking up and down your stairs at home once every other day, which could then progress to twice every other day, and so on. Or you may prefer to commit to walking in the fresh air. You could start by just walking to the first lamppost on your street and back, then increasing it to two lampposts, and so on.

As food restriction is often psychologically damaging, another goal you may wish to consider is to have a cheat (i.e. something unhealthy) on a particular day of the week. For example, if your cheat day is Saturday, then if you see something you really want during the week that you know you shouldn't have, instead of saying, 'I cannot have that anymore', which will cause you to obsess over that particular food, you can say, 'I will have that on Saturday, on my cheat day.' Often, by the time Saturday comes, you either do not want it anymore or find that it is not as amazing as you had told yourself it would be.

Winning at weight loss is about creating a new, healthier lifestyle, so commit to this in various realistic ways, rather than just going on a diet that will very likely be unsustainable.

Sugar activates the opiate receptors in our brain and affects the reward centre, which leads to compulsive behaviour, despite the negative consequences like weight gain, headaches, hormone imbalances, and more.

**Cassie Bjork R.D., L.D.,
founder of Healthy Simple Life[34]**

CASE STUDY
Kelly: Yo-yo Dieter

Kelly was the eldest of five girls, and there was a six-year gap between her and her younger sisters. She told us that she had lovely memories from those first six years when she was an only child, receiving her mum's full and constant attention. However, as each of her four sisters was born in relatively quick succession, Kelly felt that her mum was moving further and further away from her, making her feel pushed out and less important.

Talking to Kelly, we soon learned that as a child, she had identified that she would receive attention and praise if she carried out tasks to help her mum. Thus, she created the following schema: *'To receive love and attention, I have to do tasks for others.'*

With five children in the family, there was also a competition when it came to food. Kelly knew that if there were treats in the house and she didn't get to them quickly, then her sisters would. Therefore, she also created the schema: *'If I don't eat what is available quickly, I will miss out.'*

Years later, Kelly came to recognise through our time in therapy that, because she had created the behavioural schema that to obtain love and attention she had to do things for others, she had become subservient and overly eager to please. At school she would be the one who offered to help the teachers; she would stay behind after class if anything needed to be done; she would do things for her friends – and sadly, she now realised, on occasion she would be taken for granted.

When Kelly was a teenager and started dating, she felt she attracted boys who also took her for granted. This further cemented her belief that she wasn't good enough. Kelly also started to struggle with her weight and described herself as a yo-yo dieter and sugar addict.

She married when she was 22 and went on to have two children. As she was a people pleaser, she would insist on doing everything for her husband and children, yet she was quietly resentful that no one did anything for her. And because Kelly had created an unhealthy relationship with food during her childhood, even as an adult she could never just ignore treats in the house – instead, she felt compelled to eat them before anyone else did.

As we expected, Kelly confirmed that during the times when she felt she was getting the love she needed and the focus of attention was on her, such as when she first met her husband, when they got married and when they had children, she was able to control her eating far better.

We also identified that whenever Kelly felt undervalued, any diets she may have been on would come to an abrupt end; she would buy treats and unhealthy foods, and suddenly her overeating behaviours would kick in.

Identifying this pattern was a huge breakthrough moment for Kelly. Her lack of understanding of her behaviour with food and yo-yo dieting had made her feel like a failure and subsequently damaged her self-esteem.

We helped Kelly to alter her perspective of childhood events that we felt were holding her back in adulthood, particularly with regards to her self-esteem and yo-yo dieting. We began by asking her, as a mum of two children herself, whether she loved her elder child less than her second. Kelly immediately said no. We went on to ask whether her love for her elder child had diminished in any way once her second child had arrived. Kelly obviously said that she adored both her children equally. Furthermore, she agreed when we pointed it out that once her new baby arrived, her attention *was* taken up more by the younger child, but that this was due to the needs of her baby, because the baby was less capable, and never because of favouritism.

For the first time, Kelly allowed herself to 'see the situation for what it was, and not how it had felt to a six-year-old little girl'. She cried, and went on to say that she felt a little silly that she had not seen this before. It was now clear that her mum's lack of attention did not mean she loved her any less, it just meant that she knew Kelly was a capable young girl. We agreed that this was actually a compliment. We then explained that often the reason negative schemas are created is because they are based on a child's misinterpretation of events, caused by their limited life experience at the time.

Next, we looked at Kelly's eagerness to please people. It appeared that she, like many people, was willing to do far more for others than she was for herself, often to her own detriment. However, as Kelly had a schema that 'doing things for others meant love', she expected others to do the same for her, and when they did not, she misinterpreted this as meaning that '*she* wasn't good enough' and '*she* wasn't loved'.

To help positively condition this inaccurate and negative schema, we asked Kelly to consider how often she actually allowed people to do things for her. If there was a task to be done, would she let anybody else undertake it? Did she ever give people the opportunity to do things for her? She thought about this and realised that she was her own worst enemy, because despite wanting people to do things for her to show that they loved and cared for her, in reality she never allowed this to happen.

We had already established that her overeating of sweet treats at home was a result of her having to share with four other children when she was a little girl. In order to condition this schema, we asked Kelly whether her siblings still lived with her. Kelly confirmed that they did not and had not for some years. In view of her response, we then asked if there was any need for her to race to eat everything in case her siblings came round and raided her kitchen cupboards. Kelly found this funny and said no.

We also asked Kelly who was in charge of providing the treats when she was at home as a child. Kelly said her parents were. We then asked, 'Who is in control now?' Kelly realised that it was her. If she wanted more, she could have more, therefore there was no need to rush to eat all the treats, as her siblings were not going to snatch them from her anymore. To conclude our therapy session, we used our Bungee Technique (which we shared in Chapter 9, see page 167), so as to make specific sweet treats less desirable to Kelly.

Four months later, Kelly updated us by email. She told us that she had managed to maintain a healthier way of eating, making the small, slow changes we had suggested, that the extreme desire to eat sweet foods had gone and that her thoughts were no longer dominated by them as they had been before. She said that, while it was amazing, she still found it very strange that she did not crave sugary foods.

A year later, Kelly contacted us again with another update. This time, she shared with us an unexpected positive progression in her life. As she had gained control of her eating and was no longer yo-yo dieting, she had noticed that this had undoubtedly boosted her confidence. Eating healthily, exercising and losing weight felt good and was making her stronger and happier, both emotionally and physically.

This progress had also led to a positive change in the dynamics of her relationship with her husband. As Kelly had changed, she noticed that her husband had changed, too, becoming increasingly more attentive towards her. She felt that, whereas in the past she had always been eager to please, her husband was now doing far more in an effort to please her. Perhaps this was because, with her newly bolstered self-esteem, Kelly was now allowing her husband to do things for her.

CASE STUDY
Justine: Yo-yo Dieter

Justine was battling to retain a healthy weight. She had lost a great deal of weight in the past, but soon after hitting her target, she had started to gain it once more. Despite knowing how to eat and being aware of the importance of exercising, she was aware that there was an element missing in her journey.

This missing component was her failure to address a negative issue that was affecting her relationship with eating.

This was something Justine could see, but she was unsure how to resolve it.

She appeared to be a vivacious, confident, bubbly, flamboyant character, yet we felt this was a barrier that she put up to prevent people from getting too near, as a form of protection. Prior to therapy, we asked Justine to complete our timeline and questionnaire to give us an indication of things that had occurred in her life that may have contributed to her eating issues and yo-yo dieting. It was clear to see that Justine had low self-esteem. Despite never having been bullied, her opinion of herself was low because she felt she had let her parents down, particularly her mother, with whom she had been very close. On further discussion, Justine shared with us that she was gay, and although her parents knew about this, she had never actually discussed it with them as she believed they disapproved of her sexuality.

We asked what evidence Justine had to lead her to make this assumption. The only shred of potential evidence she had was a memory of having a gay friend at school, whom she thought her mother had disapproved of. She did agree, however, that in hindsight, she had assumed they had known her friend was gay, but it was possible they never knew this, and their supposed judgement may have been because the friend wasn't as studious or as committed at school as Justine was. This could have prompted her mother to worry that her friend was a distraction for her.

It was clear that Justine's inaccurate interpretation of this situation as a child had created a schema that her mum had an issue with gay people. This then resulted in Justine not wanting to talk to her parents about her sexuality. We believed this was why Justine had started to self-sabotage, using weight to make herself less attractive, thereby reducing the opportunities of falling in love, having a relationship and then having to broach the fact that she was gay with her parents. We also suggested that, as this was an emotional burden she was carrying, perhaps she was also using food to temporarily ease the pain.

We pointed out that weight gain was therefore not only sabotaging her opportunities to have a relationship; it was also another form of protection, ensuring that she was less likely to have to face her sexuality and disappoint her parents, primarily her mother. The unconscious belief that she was a disappointment to her mother was also contributing to her low self-esteem.

Knowing that she was vastly overweight and that it was affecting her health, Justine would continually yo-yo diet. She would lose some weight, which is what she wanted, but then the fear of hurting her parents would creep up like a warning light, and she would go back to protecting herself from the emotional pain with food. Furthermore, as she had inaccurately assumed that she was disappointing her mum, she would also punish herself by telling herself she did not deserve to be slim and healthy. She knew exactly how she should eat and that she should exercise, but because she had not dealt with her emotional issues and the cause of why she was self-medicating and self-sabotaging with food, she became trapped in a pattern of yo-yo dieting.

When we sat with Justine, we asked her what she thought any parent's objective is. She agreed that a parent's objective is to see their child grow up into someone who is happy and secure. We asked whether her parents, and particularly her mother, were good parents, and Justine confirmed that they were both exceptional. We asked whether her mother would want her to be happy and secure, and she confirmed that she would. We then asked whether her mother would want her to feel happy and secure regardless of anything, and whether her mother loved her unconditionally. Justine replied yes to both.

As the barriers started to come down and her inaccurate beliefs were being challenged, Justine went on to tell us stories about her mum, which showed that she had on many occasions tried to make it clear that she knew her daughter was gay and was perfectly happy with that fact. Her mum had clearly been trying to allow Justine to open up to her, without wanting to put her on the spot or make her feel uncomfortable, because she loved her so much, yet Justine never took the olive branch, as her barriers always got in the way. Her childhood schema had not allowed her to see the message her mother was trying to communicate. The fact that she didn't want to make her feel uncomfortable or put her on the spot proved just how much she loved her.

This realisation made Justine very emotional. It was a huge turning point for her: having previously tried to show us evidence that her mother was disappointed in her, she now, unprompted, began to provide us with evidence that her mother loved and accepted her. As a consequence of her inaccurate schema, Justine had previously been unable to accept this information.

After also carrying out our Mirror Technique with Justine (shared in Chapter 8, see page 148), we observed an immediate change, and her updates since have been wonderful. Not only has her relationship with her parents improved now that she feels more at ease, but she said her biggest change in behaviour has been around unhealthy food. In the past, if she had eaten anything unhealthy, she would think she had messed up her diet and would go on to eat more bad food, whereas now she was able to have a few chips or a slice of cake if she wanted some, without spiralling out of control and overeating, and she would then immediately resume healthy eating. She felt this was an incredible progression.

Justine had been freed from her past negative behavioural schema, and as a consequence, her attitude towards food and towards herself has changed.

The Not Right Now Technique

This is a great technique that you can try with food in the moment of temptation. It is what we call our Not Right Now Technique. It can be very effective to help manage cravings.

Having discovered that people visually code – people, objects and food – we found that if you alter the coding, a person's feelings towards that person, object or food can change, too, sometimes long term (we explain this idea more fully in the last chapter, in our Bungee Technique, see page 167). However, if you just want to make a temporary change and would prefer not to alter your perspective indefinitely, you can try the Not Right Now Technique.

To do this, close your eyes and imagine a picture of the food you are craving in front of you. Put your hand where you see or feel the image is positioned. You will probably notice that it is quite close to your face and looks big, bright and desirable.

Now, keeping your eyes closed, imagine yourself grabbing the image of that food and pushing it further away, as far as your hand can move it. As you do so, fade the colour and brightness from what you see. Make the image black and white, and also make it smaller.

You should now feel less tempted by that food. If you still feel tempted, repeat the process and imagine the food you want to eat floating and going even further away. You can also add an unpleasant smell to the process, too, if that helps. Imagine something you don't like, such as smelly cheese, sour milk or gone-off meat.

This is usually just a short-term solution and will not prevent you from ever wanting to eat this food again, but it's a great technique to tackle the urge in the moment, to stop you munching on things you know you shouldn't.

Checklist: Things to Do to Address Yo-yo Dieting

1 Create clear, realistic goals

Give yourself a goal, and then break that goal up into small steps so that you can see your progress and celebrate your achievements. Give yourself little rewards along the way.

2 Sleep

Get a good night's sleep. If you struggle to sleep due to the light, try black-out curtains. If you have a lot going on in your mind, write it down on a piece of paper to remove the worries from your mind. That way you can reassure yourself that everything is documented, for you to address the next morning. Avoid caffeine, sugar, alcohol and bright lights from any devices, such as your laptop or phone, before bed. When you are in bed, do not say, 'I can't sleep', as you are giving yourself the command not to sleep. Instead, with your eyes closed, say to yourself, 'I'll try to stay awake just for ten more minutes', and then relax.

3 Avoid alcohol and drugs

Alcohol and drugs will affect your ability to sleep, as well as your focus, appetite and willpower.

4 Medication

Speak with your GP about the medication you are taking and investigate any possible side effects and alternatives.

5 Hormones

Speak with your GP to enquire about blood tests for hormonal imbalance, and how you might address this. Also speak to your local health-food store to ask about natural supplements that could help.

6 Consider if you are emotionally eating

Work through your timeline and questionnaire and try to address any issues that might be affecting your eating habits. You may also wish to seek therapy via your doctor.

7 Food diary

Eat consciously by focusing on eating and nothing else. Put your knife and fork down between mouthfuls. Watching TV or being distracted promotes unconscious eating and can take away the feeling of being full, as you don't register what you have eaten. A food diary will help to make you more accountable for what you consume and when. It will also give you clues as to where and when your eating triggers may lie.

8 Healthy eating

Follow a realistic healthy-eating plan and not a diet. Do not restrict your eating; instead, consider healthy versions of the foods and dishes you enjoy. Think about how you can adapt your favourite meals to make them healthier.

9 Stress

Consider ways you can reduce or resolve new stresses in your life. You may find that talking to a friend helps. Also keeping a diary, exercising, doing yoga, listening to music or writing a problem on a Post-it note and placing it in front of you so that you can address just one issue at a time can all be very helpful.

10 Our techniques

Try applying our Bungee Technique (see page 167) to foods that sabotage your success, and the Not Right Now Technique (see page 189) before succumbing to an unhealthy option.

11

Food Phobias and Anxiety Around Food

Fussy eating habits affect more than eight in ten families across the UK, bringing with it a significant emotional burden on family life. 60 per cent of parents said fussy eating was a cause of frustration, one-third said it made them worry and 27 per cent reported the situation led to feelings of anxiety and powerlessness.

Online survey results from over 1,000 parents, Abbott Healthcare[35]

Everyone is aware that healthy eating goes hand in hand with having a healthy body and being a healthy weight. However, for some people who have sought our help, the prospect of eating fruit or vegetables has been absolutely impossible, as they experience anxiety, fear and nausea when faced with such foods.

Food phobias, food aversion, avoidant restrictive food intake disorder (ARFID), food dislikes, food neophobia, picky eating, fussy eating, cibophobia and selective eating disorder are all terms used to describe someone who is averse to eating particular foods. Those suffering with any of these conditions can especially struggle if their condition relates to foods that are considered healthy. We have encountered many individuals over the years who have only been able to eat chips, bread and chocolate, others who could only eat chicken, bacon and chips and others who would experience a panic attack when attempting to eat vegetables or anything green.

With that in mind, we wanted to address any food aversions or phobias you may have that could be hindering your healthy eating.

What Stops You Eating Healthily?

Every behaviour you have is as a consequence of learning. This learning comes from a life experience you have had or from copying someone else's behaviour. Both are very much based on your personal interpretation of the event at the time or who/what you were copying.

For example, you and a friend could be involved in an argument over the very same event, because you both have an individual interpretation of that event based on your own personal experiences. You might think your friend at school should share her sweets. Because you have siblings, you will have been taught and perhaps made to share, whereas your friend may be an only child, and therefore sharing was not a significant part of their learning.

Copying behaviour is similarly based on how you perceive a situation. For example, you may see your mother avoid cats, and as a consequence you may develop a phobia of cats, assuming that her avoidance must be due to cats being dangerous. However, the truth could be that your mother does not have a phobia – in fact, she tries to avoid them because she has an allergy to them. This misinterpretation and *misunderstanding* could completely shape your life, leaving you filled with fear and anxiety at the sight of a cat and unable to visit friends' homes just in case they have one.

Every food-related phobia and aversion that we have encountered in our clinic has been as a result of this kind of *misunderstanding*, where behaviours, opinions and attitudes have been learned on the basis of misinterpretation, and it has a huge bearing on what the person eats and their overall relationship with food.

There are a numerous reasons why you might develop a phobia, aversion or revulsion to healthy foods and feel unable to eat them. These include:

Unpleasant childhood experience

Unpleasant or traumatic childhood experiences often lead to food aversion. A common example is choking on a certain food as a child. Rather than realising that this was due to not chewing the food enough, or being distracted or startled while eating, the specific food or all similar foods are blamed and avoided in the future, in an effort to protect yourself from the offending food.

For some, all foods can become an issue after a choking incident, resulting in only being able to consume liquids thereafter, which can lead to weight loss and even malnutrition. In these cases, the person blames all food, and loses confidence in their ability to swallow, instead of appreciating that they have been able to swallow from the moment they were born and that, despite having choked briefly, they survived. Once the person realises that not only did they survive but that it wasn't the food's fault, they can entirely condition the schema and change their resulting behaviours.

Vomiting or a severe stomach upset after eating a certain food can also lead to avoidance of that food or associated foods. Again, in that situation, if the item was not cooked correctly, the solution should be to avoid food prepared by that person or establishment. Yet in the moment, the unpleasant situation is often linked to the food itself, and therefore the food is avoided. Equally, if a child notices a particular food in vomit, such as carrots, a negative association can be made with carrots from that day forth.

Poor example

As children copy behaviour, those who sit together around a table for their evening meal with their parents tend to have a better relationship with food.

If a positive parental example is not set, this can lead to children avoiding or believing they do not like healthy foods. Inexperience of new foods can also lead to caution or anxiety around them.

First experience

A scientific study has found that we start to form impressions of a person in less than one-tenth of a second.[36] With that in mind, the saying 'You only get one chance to make a first impression' can be very significant in the context of what we are eating. If you gained a poor first impression of certain healthy foods as a child because they were cooked or presented badly, this can result in food avoidance and an unfair dislike based on the person who prepared your initial experience.

We have found that school dinners during childhood are a significant contributor to a poor first experience, as they often included bland, overcooked vegetables. Worst still, if you were forced to eat those vegetables and were punished or chastised if you did not, this could condition vegetables in your mind as something to be avoided as soon as you are in charge of your own diet.

Emetophobia

Emetophobia is a fear of vomiting, which can manifest as an avoidance of anything that could potentially lead to a sickness bug or vomiting. If someone with emetophobia hears of anyone being sick after eating a certain food or thinks there is any possibility that a food could make them sick, they will then avoid it at all costs.

These tend to be foods such as chicken, which can cause tummy upsets if not cooked thoroughly, but we have also encountered people who will not eat salad, fruit or anything uncooked, as they worry that it is not clean enough or, unless overcooked, it could be contaminated.

Over-accommodating parent or carer

The second-most common cause we have encountered for food avoidance, after having had a negative or traumatic experience with foods, is an over-accommodating parent.

When a parent has allowed their little one to dictate their own diet, that child will often grow up to be inexperienced and nervous about new foods. This could be because they were picky as a child, and therefore their parent felt relieved at whatever their child would eat, as they worried that they would become sick if they didn't eat. Often parents who worry about their child's eating are told by their doctor to give their child whatever they are happy to eat, as they are likely to grow out of their picky-eating phase.

Some parents also make assumptions about their child's likes or dislikes, and in so doing inadvertently instruct their child not to like certain foods or textures. If, for example, a child refuses to eat or spits out certain foods or vomits after a meal, the parent may well assume that this first experience equates to their child not liking or being able to eat that food. The child then hears their parent telling them, 'You don't like that', and therefore a behavioural schema is created by the child towards that food, unless it is challenged.

In defence of parents, however, children do not come with an instruction manual, and parents can only ever strive to do their best. If they are not given any direction on how to introduce new foods to their child as they grow, this can lead to very limited eating for that child in adulthood, which is why many of the people we help in our clinic with food-aversion issues tend to eat only childish foods, such as chicken nuggets, chips, yoghurt, fromage frais, chocolate and toast.

My mum always told me I didn't like tomatoes, and so I told everyone I hated them. I couldn't even try and swallow anything with tomato in it. No ketchup, no bolognaise or chilli sauces. It wasn't until I was in my late teens, at university, under the influence of a few too many wines, that I ate what I thought was a mini quiche, which turned out to be pizza with a tomato base, and I loved it! Suffice it to say, I am now a tomato fan – ha ha!

Lydia

Texture

A parent is often eager to start weaning their child off milk and onto solid foods, as it not only aids their growth, but is also often deemed to contribute to a better night's sleep.

However, in an effort to end those night-time feeds, a hasty parent could potentially cause a poor first experience for the baby, giving them solids before they are ready and thus creating a negative association with solid foods.

Similarly, a toddler who observes their parent panicking about things being too big or lumpy for their little one to swallow or the possibility of their child choking can develop negative associations with food – particularly food of those kinds of textures.

CASE STUDY
Tina: Fruit and Vegetable Phobia

For someone quite short in stature, to be 16 stone (224lb/102kg) in weight is significant, and for Tina it had resulted in her having diabetes, high blood pressure and sleep apnoea.

Tina told us that she believed she had an issue with weight because she had a severe phobia of all fruit and vegetables (except French fries) and so could not eat well. It was so severe that she could not even have any sauces or gravy on her food, just in case they contained any water that vegetables had been cooked in. Tina also told us that there were many occasions when she, her husband and two children would go out as a family, but they would have to eat in two different places in the same retail park. Her husband and children would eat in a restaurant, whereas Tina would eat at a fast-food chain so that she could ensure she was just eating fried chicken or fries.

Tina's diet consisted of fried chicken, bread, fries, cake, chocolate and sweets. She also ate a lot of dairy products, especially high-fat cheese and butter. She had not eaten any fruits or vegetables whatsoever since childhood. She was repulsed by them. She couldn't bear to be anywhere near them, and the thought of letting them pass her lips in any form made her incredibly anxious.

Tina knew she was not setting a good example to her children, and that it was also causing issues in her marriage. Not only was she unhealthy, unfit and unable to take part in family activities, but she was also the cause of a big division within her family. Tina was convinced that most restaurants would contaminate food with fruit or vegetables, and because of this she was unable to socialise with friends or family or go to any restaurants for dinner. Her world was becoming smaller as the years were passing. The restrictions she was putting on herself and the way she was adapting her life to accommodate her phobia was getting worse, as was her health and weight.

Tina truly believed she was a lost cause, that her issues around food were hers for life and that they would eventually take her life!

We explained to Tina that nobody is born with any fears, likes or dislikes concerning foods, and that all our behaviours are learned as a result of our life experiences. Tina was fairly confident that she knew the origin of her fear of fruit and vegetables, and she went on to share the distressing details of her childhood.

Tina had attended a very strict school. She vividly remembers having lunch in the school hall, where the headmistress would shout at the children if they did not clear their plates. One day, early on in her school career, Tina did not feel very well but was too shy to mention this to her teacher. She had sat down to eat her lunch of meat, vegetables and potatoes, and confirmed that, at that point, she had no fear of eating the vegetables on her plate. She would normally have eaten her lunch, but on this particular day, as she was feeling unwell, she only picked at it.

When she could eat no more, she began to carry her plate to the trays where the children would stack their plates, but the headmistress spotted her and, in front of everyone, bellowed at her to sit back down and finish her lunch. Tina felt embarrassed and scared, and although she attempted to eat a little more, she couldn't, and tried to explain that she did not feel very well and did not want it.

The headmistress had different ideas, however, and started to feed Tina until she vomited all over the table and her plate. In this heightened state of stress, she looked down at her plate and recalled seeing what looked like gravy with little bits of green broccoli pieces in it. The whole situation, including the smell, had an enormous impact on her, right up until the day we met her.

Tina had created an aversion to eating vegetables, which she had associated with her memory of vomiting ever since that day in the dining hall. As is always the case with phobias, rather than rationalise what had happened – that the headmistress had been wrong and had caused her issues with food – Tina had unconsciously attributed her feelings of upset, embarrassment and illness to the vegetables, creating a negative schema. She quite literally blamed the vegetables for the headmistress's inexcusable behaviour.

Sadly, Tina's issues in school did not stop there. As she now had an aversion to eating vegetables and to eating at school, the headmistress forced her to eat lunch in her office every day, intimidating her by standing over her until she was finished. Her fear therefore grew, becoming worse and worse, so that by the time she left school, she never wanted to eat vegetables ever again. The only foods she felt safe around were those she would not normally have at school, which included the things she ate now, such as fried chicken, chips, crisps, chocolate and sweets.

When we met with Tina, her fear and aversion to fruit and vegetables were evident – we were unable to have any fruit in the room.

As our therapy is evidential, part of our process often involves showing the person the item they feel uncomfortable with, even if it is just a photograph, for the purposes of a before and after, so that they can immediately feel the difference. This was not something Tina could participate in, however, as her aversion was so extreme.

Due to the extent of her fear, we wanted to see Tina over two sessions, and as her fear of fruit was slightly less severe than her fear of vegetables, we agreed to start our first session talking about fruit.

We spoke about the incident at school and helped Tina to understand why she had created the aversion around fruit and vegetables. We asked her to tell us how she thought the fruit or vegetables had been responsible for her feeling humiliated, embarrassed or scared. Her instant reaction was to tell us they had made her sick. We then asked whether she had already felt sick that day when she sat down for lunch, prior to eating anything. She thought for a moment, and then said she came to lunch already feeling unwell. We therefore asked whether she had already eaten any fruit or vegetables prior to coming to lunch. She would probably have just had her breakfast, she said, which would have been cereal or porridge. So we asked again how fruit or vegetables were to blame for what happened.

Tina started to smile and told us that she knew what we were saying and knew where we were going with it. She now agreed with us that, in fact, the fruit and vegetables did not cause her to be sick.

To encourage Tina to smile a little more, and also to help her see the situation for what it was and not how it had felt to her as a little girl, we said, 'All those years, your headmistress dealt with you badly, and ever since you have been blaming fruit and vegetables for making you sick when they had nothing to do with it – you've been giving them a really rough ride!'

Tina smiled and said, 'It seems that way, doesn't it?'

We then carried out our Bungee Technique (see Chapter 9, page 167) in reverse to bring fruit closer in her coded position to make it more desirable to her. We then brought a little bit of apple for Tina to try. Although a little apprehensive – after all, it had been over 40 years since fruit or anything green had passed her lips – Tina admitted that she felt no fear associated with it, which felt strange.

She nibbled on the apple and told us that it was 'quite nice' and 'refreshing'. From there, we offered her pieces of strawberry, peach, grape, orange and melon. We were all delighted with how far she had come, and that she had tried and even enjoyed them all.

In her second session, there were two things we wanted to address. The first was to make vegetables more desirable to her by, and the second was to make chocolate and sweets less desirable to help her tackle her diabetes and obesity. To treat both of these issues, we repeated the Bungee Technique.

In that second session, not only did Tina eat vegetables and broccoli, which had always been her biggest nemesis, she even tried a piece of *raw* broccoli, which we felt was the biggest milestone yet in her journey.

We were thrilled to hear from Tina as the months went by that she had begun to eat a normal, balanced diet, had reduced her intake of sweet treats and was losing weight. Family days out were now true family days out, as they all went to the same restaurant!

Tina's case was incredibly rewarding, because we know that had she not made dramatic changes to her diet, the consequences for her could have been catastrophic. To know that she was now ingesting good foods full of vitamins and minerals, and that she was now able to spend time with her family eating together, gave us both so much joy. Although it was some years ago that we saw Tina, we have never forgotten her or the difference we saw in her after our therapy sessions.

Thanks so much, Nik and Eva, for helping me to eat fruit and vegetables. This is beyond life-changing and I'm still in so much shock that I can eat them . . . and even more shocking – I actually like them!

Tina

CASE STUDY
Daniel: Food Aversion

Daniel was a 20-year-old professional rugby player who would have had a promising career ahead of him if it weren't for some health issues with his knees, which forced him to medically retire. Daniel was absolutely devastated, but he knew that his health problems had arisen entirely because of his poor diet.

For as long as Daniel could remember, he had only ever eaten chips, chocolate and yoghurt; he could not eat anything else. He told us that he would go to restaurants with his girlfriend and pretend that his mum, not knowing he was going out for a meal, had made him food before he left, and he had felt obliged to eat it because he didn't want to let her down. He told his girlfriend that he didn't want to let her down either, so she should order a meal and he would just order a plate of chips.

Daniel had spoken about his food issues with his mother, and she had told him that, when he was a child, he was a fussy eater. She had taken him to see the family doctor, who had assured her that as long as he was eating something, she shouldn't push him, as he would soon grow out of it.

Evidently, Daniel never did grow out of it, though, and had never tried any other foods. And now, the fact that he had eaten hardly anything other than chips had taken its toll on Daniel's body and was jeopardising his health and his career. Daniel felt he needed to take some action. He had tried hypnotherapy and a talking therapy, both with little success, and therefore asked if there was anything we could do to help.

We wanted to know a little bit more about Daniel's life and his childhood. It appeared that his upbringing was lovely, with no major traumas – on the contrary, he told us he was a very happy, spoilt little boy and that his mum would do absolutely anything for him.

As we talked further, it became apparent that the only reason Daniel had not eaten anything other than chips, chocolate and yoghurt was because that was what he had liked as a child. He assumed that his attitude must have been, 'What's the point of eating anything else when I like what I like?' Furthermore, as a little boy, he knew he could get away with not eating anything else, as his mum was so kind and accommodating.

As his behavioural schema around new foods had been established at a young age, he never questioned it when he heard his mother telling people how he would not eat anything except chips, chocolate and yoghurt. He grew up believing he did not like anything else and that he could not eat anything else. He had imposed a block on trying new foods but had never been curious about the root cause behind it.

We pointed out that, just as his mum had told him he was called Daniel, which he had never questioned, she had also told him that he was a fussy eater, which he had also never questioned.

When we started to dissect what had actually happened with Daniel, it appeared that he had likely manipulated his mum to give him exactly what he wanted to eat, and this habit had just grown out of control, hence why he found himself in his current situation.

This realisation alone created a shift in Daniel, although he was not yet ready to try new foods. We needed to provide more evidence to condition Daniel's schema, and so we pointed out that at the age of 20, he was in fact being dictated to by a little boy of maybe two or three years of age – that little boy, of course, being him.

Daniel agreed, and went on to say that there was nothing

stopping him from trying new things except himself. He completely understood how this had probably come about.

We assured Daniel that we would not ask him to do anything dangerous or detrimental to his health, but also asked if he trusted us. Daniel said he did and that was why he was with us. We added, 'As a 20-year-old man, you can either choose to take control of your life and what you eat, or allow yourself to be controlled by a child.' Daniel confirmed that he wanted to take control of his eating as an adult.

We pointed out that he had actually been controlling everything from the age of two or three. Back then, he had made the right choices for a three-year-old, but they were not the right choices for a man. He had also chosen to play with toys at that age, so by his logic, if he wanted to still listen to himself as a child, should he not carry on playing with toys? Daniel laughed. We asked why he no longer played with toys, and his response was: 'Because I've grown up – or at least I thought I had.'

Before we could say any more, Daniel acknowledged that it was time to make an adult choice. We asked him if he was ready to try some new foods, and he agreed that he was.

Slowly, we introduced Daniel to new foods and the block was removed. The only thing that remained was a lack of knowledge about the textures and tastes he was about to experience. We wanted Daniel to try as many foods as possible before he left us to build his confidence and prove to himself that his previous belief was untrue – he *was* able to try anything. During our session he tried chicken, chicken nuggets, mashed potato, peas, carrots, broccoli, banana, grapes, peaches and toast. Something we had not factored in was Daniel's lack of experience with cutlery, as he had never had to use a knife and fork together before, but it was still so lovely to watch his reactions to these new foods and see his appreciation of the ones he enjoyed. He could not believe he had been missing out on so many great things for so long.

Daniel's mum came to collect him at the end of our session, and we were all very proud to show her that he was now able to eat the chicken, mashed potato and vegetables that we had prepared. It was so emotional to see his mum cry with happiness and relief.

We asked his mum whether she had felt responsible for his food aversions. She confirmed that she had carried a huge weight of guilt on her shoulders for years. She even said in front of Daniel that she blamed herself for him losing out on the career he had always wanted as a rugby player. We were so pleased that she had come to collect him, as it meant that we could help them both, and Daniel could let his mum know that it was okay – he did not blame her. We pointed out to her that, on the contrary, by allowing him to eat what he wanted, she had actually been trying to show how much she loved him. We also reminded her that she had taken professional advice from a doctor, who had told her that it was okay for Daniel to just eat what he wanted.

Daniel's case was a really interesting one for us, and we were absolutely thrilled to have helped a young man on his journey towards health, strength and recovery.

Opting for Healthier Foods

If you struggle with a food phobia, an aversion or with healthy eating generally, we hope that this chapter and its case studies have given you some food for thought as to the origins of your feelings towards certain foods. In summary, here are some suggestions that might help:

1   The first step to fixing anything is to understand what has gone wrong in the first place. Look through your timeline to see if you can find the origin of your aversion. Did you have a traumatic experience? If so, consider whether the

food was really to blame. Was it the food or was it the cook?

2　Consider your role models and any copied behaviours you may have taken on. If this applies, understand that you are using someone else's palate to dictate your eating patterns. Would you allow that person to dictate what you wear? Who you date? Who you socialise with? What you drink? Where you work? Your hobbies? If not, why not? Apply your response to this answer to your pattern of eating, too.

3　Is your aversion orientated around texture? If so, how might this have occurred? Could it be a result of parental weaning? Something you once ate that was badly cooked? A parental reaction to you possibly choking on something as a child? If so, how was the texture to blame for this? Has your swallowing reflex ever let you down? Even if you had a choking experience, what actually happened other than a few moments of discomfort?

4　Try the Bungee Technique (see page 167) in reverse to bring healthy foods you dislike towards you. See them closer and make their colours brighter.

5　Think of all the new things you have ever tried, such as driving or a new job, and notice that when we try anything new a feeling of apprehension exists. Do not misinterpret this natural apprehension as fear or an inability to try something new.

6　If your aversion has existed from childhood, ask yourself when you would ever take the advice of a child on important life decisions.

7   Try new foods in the tastiest, most enjoyable way possible. Give yourself the best first experience by trying new foods at a restaurant with a friend. Not only will turning the challenge into a pleasant event provide a distraction, but you are more likely to go ahead with it if you have someone else there to encourage you, support you and praise you.

8   Do not feel under pressure; there will be some new foods you like and some you don't. Very few people love every type of food, and that is okay.

9   Remember that, if you didn't like a certain type of food the first time you tried it, that could mean you just didn't like the way it was cooked. There are so many different ways to cook the same food – many people don't even like their favourite food when it is cooked in certain ways.

10 Appreciate that you are not choosing to eat healthy foods to punish yourself in any way – you are eating to improve your life and your health.

12

Changing Your Eating and Moving Habits for Good

I'm so grateful for what you have done for me. I'm living my life now and I'm hopeful about the future. I've lost weight and I'm on my way to achieving two of my goals of gaining a counselling qualification and taking part in the London Marathon. Thanks for everything.

Melissa

The Past

As you will now know, we believe that all behaviours are learned, and that issues from your past can go on to affect your behaviours in the present. In Chapter 6 (see page 92), we talked about some possible issues that could be contributing to your unhealthy relationship with food. These included:

- **Self-medicating**
- **Protection**
- **Comfort**
- **Heartbreak**
- **Loneliness**
- **Boredom**

- **Emulation/copying behaviour/needing to belong**
- **Attention/friendship**
- **Low self-esteem due to being bullied, humiliated or embarrassed**

We would now like you to start addressing your own issues and conditioning your negative schemas. It is important to deal with just one at a time. The way to condition a past negative schema is to positively alter your perspective on the painful event that created it. So it is now time to use your timeline and questionnaire, together with the evidence you collated in Chapter 6, to consider all the negative, embarrassing, upsetting, painful, limiting events that have occurred in your life, as well as the examples set to you in relation to eating. Use a highlighter pen to mark everything you think could be relevant.

We will give you some suggestions on how to positively upgrade your schemas, but the timeline will also help you take a huge leap forward. If you are seeking therapy, you will also now have a list you can share with your therapist of the areas you would like to address.

After highlighting all potential events in your timeline and questionnaire, look at each one and, if you have not done so already, score how you feel about them. Zero would suggest you have no negative feelings about it whatsoever, while ten denotes a high level of discomfort. Scoring your emotions on a scale of disturbance or discomfort helps you to monitor your progress.

Thank you . . . very insightful and informative . . . I realise my schemas are rooted in abandonment, embarrassment and anger due to previously having my choices taken from me. You are very kind and generous people and it was a pleasure to meet you. Best wishes.

Stephen

Conditioning Your Schema

To help you address the negative events you have identified in your timeline and questionnaire, we would like to share some tips on how best to tackle the process of conditioning and upgrading your schemas.

To try to reduce the negative effects of any painful or upsetting memories, it is important to find something positive in them to help you feel better. Given that thoughts create feelings, feelings create actions and actions create habits, the way to eliminate your negative behaviours is to condition your thoughts, as this will trigger a chain reaction, subsequently changing your feelings, actions and habits, too. This may involve acknowledging that you have learnt something new from the experience, that the event made you stronger, kinder or more empathetic or that it enabled you to help somebody else as a result of what you have been through.

As previously mentioned, do also consider that if the event has been and gone, you are no longer a victim of that event; you survived it. And you can change your emotional attachment to it by accepting that it was never personal to you. Appreciate that you have already survived your very worst day, and that was because of you, not your weight.

With regards to the issues that may be standing in the way of you achieving your weight-loss goals, here are some points to consider. Not all will apply to you, but all are worth considering when working through your timeline.

Addressing Negative Events on Your Timeline

If you once felt that being big kept you safe, does that still apply today? If the person you were protecting yourself from is no longer in your life, acknowledge that your task is completed and you no longer need to be big to protect yourself.

If the person you are protecting yourself from is still in your life and is continuing to hurt you, please speak to someone in confidence. There are numerous charities you can anonymously call, who want you to call them for their support. Also consider the following: can you avoid this person? Can you walk away? Can other family members help you or mediate a conversation with them? Can you stand up to them without being aggressive to show them you are no longer willing to accept their behaviour? This can be very empowering for you and can make them realise that you are in control of your life.

If you used your weight to hide away, did that work for you? Was it really successful? Did it make you happy? If you are hiding yourself away now, consider how much value you could give to a friend or someone else who needs a friend. It is important for you to share your friendship and kindness with others. In fact, hiding yourself away could be considered selfish, as you could be adding value and joy to someone else's life.

If you use weight to avoid getting into a relationship, because you have had your heart broken in the past and worry that all relationships will cause you emotional pain, consider that this is like blaming a stranger for something they did not do. You need to shift the blame from relationships to the partner who broke your heart, as that person does not represent all relationships. Think of all the years you survived perfectly well before you ever knew that person and be reassured that you will again.

If you have had your heart broken and you want that person back, consider whether eating could ever repair your relationship. Would being overweight make it more or less likely?

If someone broke your heart and you do not want them back, imagine if you were to bump into them today. Would you feel better or worse? Consider that question again, if you were to bump into them looking fit and healthy – the best you have ever looked. Which feels better and why? If looking great would make you feel strong and empowered, use this image as a motivator to encourage you to be your very best.

If you use weight to hide who you really are, remember that those who love you do so unconditionally, not for who you want to date, what you want to wear, because of the car you drive or the hobbies you have. They love you for being you.

Perhaps you use your weight as a persona. Do you believe it gives you a personality and something to hide behind? If so, you should carry out our Mirror Technique (see page 148) to help build your self-esteem.

If you have ever felt rejected by a parent, partner or friend and consequently eat for comfort, consider that we are all individual and have a different definition of what being a parent, partner or friend entails. Their behaviour towards you is likely due to their own personal life experiences and not because of you. They may have a schema that being loved and giving love can lead to pain, perhaps because they themselves were once rejected, so they are protecting themselves from this potential pain by pushing you away. This does not justify their behaviour, but it could explain it and confirm that it was not intended to hurt you.

To address this hurt, make a list of everyone who loves you or has loved you (include pets, friends, children and even ex-partners). Think about why they loved you. Would you give your love to anyone who did not deserve it? Does anyone give love away freely or does it have to be earned? Remember that if you have ever been loved, it is because you are lovable.

Have you lost someone? Do you struggle with grief? If so, know that this is a process and you will never forget that person. It is important to hold on to the life they had and not their death. Remember all the times you laughed and had fun together. Talk about them with loved ones. Talk to them when you are alone. Make a promise to them to concentrate on your health so that, as their ambassador on this earth, you will keep their memory alive and enjoy health and adventures in their honour.

If your weight issues are a consequence of emulating a parent, partner, sibling or friend, ask yourself whether overeating has worked for them. Has it improved their life? If not, why not? Would you being big make them feel they have been a positive or negative role model? How might that make them feel? Would the person you are emulating love you any less if you were to lose weight? If not, why not? If you were to lose weight, could that help motivate the person you are emulating to lose weight, too? If so, how would that make you feel?

If you are copying a parent's negative behaviours around weight, realise that the behaviour does not belong to you.

You are now in control. Do they have any other negative habits that you dislike? Why do you not like it? Why do you not do the same? Now apply the same process to your emulation of their eating habits.

If you have yo-yo dieted or copied the behaviour of a yo-yo dieter and punish yourself for having 'failed' restrictive diets, realise that these diets can never work long term, as they are unrealistic. Know that everyone who embarks on them will likely have the same result. Remember, also, that when you were a baby learning to walk, you fell many times, but this did not put you off walking; you merely had to perfect being able to walk. Similarly, you have not failed with weight loss; you are working to perfect the act of healthy eating.

Do you live with someone who is overweight? People like people who are like themselves, so be careful not to become overweight like them – work on being slim together. Do you do absolutely everything they do? If not, why not? If this is a friend who encourages overeating and makes it seem acceptable, how does this benefit your life? How does it benefit theirs? Would it help or hinder them if you made healthier, more positive changes to your diet? Would your encouragement and positive changes help you both to live longer and better? Consider the value of the gift of health. Can you persuade this person to join you on the journey? If not, appreciate all the things you have achieved in your own right.

If you talk to someone regularly about eating, who is that person and how do your conversations encourage you both to get fit and heathy? If they don't, you must either make a decision to talk about something else or ask them to talk to you while taking a walk or going to the gym, to give you a more positive commonality.

If you have endured an abusive relationship, know that the abusive partner will have been abusive to others and will continue to be in the future; it was not personal to you, as it was the abuser who had the issue and they would consequently display the same behaviour with anyone they were with.

The same applies if you have been bullied or made to feel worthless. Is that person in your life now? Why would you want to listen to them? Who is responsible for what you eat? If they made you feel bad, and now overeating makes you feel bad, you are continuing to bully yourself where they left off. And being unkind or making anyone (even yourself) feel bad is not in your nature.

Pity your bully. For a person to be toxic suggests they have come from a toxic environment themselves. A bully bullies, so although it felt terrible to you, know that it was not personal. A bully will have bullied others and will continue to bully others in the future until they address their own issues. Bullies generally have low self-esteem and will bully to elevate their own status. Furthermore, they tend to only bully people whose qualities outshine their own! Please appreciate, therefore, that you are amazing and your shine dazzled them.

If the memory of a past bully continues to make you feel bad or uncomfortable, you can also try our Bungee Technique (see page 167) to move your perception of their image further away from you so as to distance yourself from them emotionally.

Finally, as you positively challenge each past negative life event, remember to only work on one at a time. When you have done that, revisit each one to re-score your emotional response from zero to ten. We hope that you have been able to positively alter your perspective on each event, but if you are still struggling then consider speaking to a trusted friend or therapist who might be able to offer you more evidence and suggestions on how to view your past life events in a more positive light, helping you to sever that negative emotional tie.

Still no chocolate. I really can't believe it! When I look at it I feel nothing, like it's something I've never tried. I can't thank you guys enough for all your support and compassion you show everyone.

Sarah

New Habits for a New You

Fully engage with and enjoy your food

If you eat while watching television, looking at social media or being distracted in any way, you are eating unconsciously. This results in not actually acknowledging everything you have eaten and therefore not being aware when you are full.

Learn to eat without distraction and focus entirely on your food – every mouthful. Really enjoy it. Slow your mealtime down by putting your cutlery down after each mouthful and chew fully to appreciate the taste of your food. This has several benefits. First, you will eat less. Second, what you do eat you will enjoy more. And third, your digestive system will have less work to do.

Don't starve

If you feel hungry, first drink a glass of water. Then, if you still feel hungry 20 minutes later, eat something.

Buy smaller plates

Most of us were taught when we were little that it's good manners to clear our plate, and big plates usually mean big portions. Buying smaller plates will naturally help you fill them with smaller portions, but also don't be afraid to leave something. It might feel very alien to do this, but leaving even a small amount will help you create better habits around food, instead of being driven by other people's old commands.

If you feel full, stop eating

While this sounds like common sense, as mentioned above, if you have been taught to clear your plate, you probably will.

On average our stomachs can hold up to 4 litres, with the feeling of being full resulting from messages sent from the stomach to the brain and chemicals released in our brain when we have had enough to eat and drink. However, an issue can arise if eating too quickly, as your food hasn't had time to be processed. Overeating can occur when some of the glucose in the food is absorbed before the fullness hormones are released, a process that can take up to 20 minutes. A study published by the *Journal of Clinical Endocrinology & Metabolism* found that slowing down our pace of eating encourages the release of the hormones that tell your brain you are indeed full, and therefore can stop eating.[37]

A slower pace of eating therefore is paramount to your weight-loss success. Take your time and enjoy every bite of your meal. It is then a good idea to wait at least 20 minutes before deciding if you need more. This tactic can be particularly helpful if you are eating out, although having dinner with friends and chatting naturally slows down your pace of eating and is therefore far more beneficial to eating alone. Remember, also, that as soon as you do feel full, you should stop eating and leave whatever is left on your plate.

Top tips for healthy eating

* Remember that you were not born overweight, and you do not have to live that way.

* Identify and work on the reason(s) why you struggle to lose weight using your timeline and questionnaire (see page 12).

* Keep a food diary (see page 78).

* Drink more water and carry a bottle of water with you at all times (see page 87).

* Eat food in its natural state i.e. choose foods without artificial flavourings.

* Use the nutrition panel on food packets to compare products, which will help you make informed, healthier choices.

* Put more good foods into your body, such as vegetables.

* Exercise or move at least three times per week, for a minimum of 25 minutes.

* When exercising, get out of breath and use weights.

* Avoid animal fats, lard, palm oil and saturated fats.

* Grill, roast or poach meats and fish, as opposed to frying.

* Avoid chicken or fish in a coating (breadcrumbs or batter).

* Invest in a George Foreman-type grill, slow-cooker and non-stick frying pan.

* Use fresh herbs, pepper and natural seasonings for flavour.

* Fry in water or spray oil only.

* Prepare a large pan of vegetable soup by frying onions, garlic and vegetables, then adding water, a vegetable stock cube and some fresh herbs, then liquidising. Have this as a starter to fill you up, and during the day when you're hungry.

* Exfoliate! Get your circulation going!

* Eat consciously and slowly. Engage with your meal and avoid distractions. Watching television while you eat, for example, will prevent this and encourage you to eat more (see page 223).

* Do your grocery shopping online to prevent the in-store temptations.

* Prepare dinner in advance to prevent snacking. Slow-cookers are great for this purpose.

* Do not eat carbohydrates after 7 p.m.

* Get a minimum of eight hours' sleep each night (see page 59).

* Buy smaller plates (see page 224).

* Avoid cheese, butter, pastry and pies.

* Avoid animal skin, rind and fats.

* Use kitchen roll to absorb or gently squeeze out excess fat from foods.

* Use kitchen roll to absorb fat from the top of casseroles, curries and sauces.

* Warm oil in a pan, then wipe the excess oil away with kitchen roll.

* Make mashed potatoes with soya milk or almond milk and a little avocado for a creamy taste.

* Fill up your dinner plate with vegetables.

* If you have a sweet tooth, prepare a fruit platter before dinner to have as a dessert.

* If you're desperate for a sweet treat, egg whites with a sugar replacement makes a great meringue, which can be eaten with fresh berries and a little soya or coconut yoghurt.

* Try gluten-free pasta, brown rice, brown rice noodles and sweet potatoes as alternatives to other starchy carbohydrates.

* Avoid alcohol.

* Use low-fat salad dressing or a light drizzle of your own home-made dressing, made with equal parts extra-virgin olive oil and balsamic vinegar, plus seasoning.

* Do not diet but DO eat to be healthy.

* Do not tell yourself you can't have something; save it for your 'cheat day' (see page 180).

* Substitute your high-fat, high-sugar, high-starch favourites with healthier alternatives. For example, use avocado as a substitute for butter.

* Consider joining a weight-loss club or group to keep you motivated and accountable until your new healthy way of eating becomes habitual and effortless.

Just wanted to say THANK YOU! Since Friday I have not stopped smiling and it's all down to the time you took with me to resolve my issues. I cannot thank you enough! Once again, a very big thank you for being you, and for your kindness.

Tiffany

Healthier Alternatives

I still have not eaten chocolate or crisps since I went to a workshop a couple of years ago.

Carole Anne

If you restrict yourself, your mind will persistently remind you of what you should not or cannot have, making you want it all the more. It is therefore far more beneficial to consider a healthier alternative – which can even be a fun challenge. Here are some of our suggestions:

* Try non-dairy alternatives, such as almond-, oat-, coconut- and soya-based products.

* Try turkey bacon as opposed to pork bacon.

* Switch to a lower fat, lean turkey, chicken or Quorn mince. Some types contain up to 20 per cent fat so always read the label.

* Have healthy snacks available, such as fruit, vegetable sticks, raisins, rice cakes, low-fat soya or coconut yoghurts, gluten-free or rye crackers or gluten-free bread for toast, lightly spread with honey, avocado or nut butter. Dried fruit and unsalted nuts are also good, but watch your portion size as, though they are healthy, they are quite high in calories.

* Choose tomato- or vegetable-based sauces over cream- or cheese-based ones.

* The best way to overcome a sweet tooth is to eat less sweet food. The less sugar you eat, the less you will crave it.

* Try our fat-free, sugar-free, gluten-free treats, cakes and recipes (see Chapter 14).

* Instead of having sandwiches for lunch, try a gluten-free wrap with salad, avocado, tuna, turkey ham, chicken or hummus.

Eating Out or Ordering In

Being healthy is far easier today than it has ever been, with more restaurants now offering healthier options, but to support your weight-loss goals, eating out and ordering in should still be considered a treat, not a lifestyle. For when you are eating from a menu, however, here are some suggestions to help you make healthier choices:

* Most restaurants share their menu online, so make your healthy choices before you arrive. This will help combat the temptation caused by what your friends or family are ordering.

* When ordering, be sure to remind the server that you do not want any butter on your vegetables.

* At an Indian restaurant, choose tomato-based curries like tandoori and madras instead of dairy-based dishes such as korma or pasanda.

* Have plain rice and chapati instead of pilau rice and naan.

* Have thick, straight-cut chips or wedges instead of French fries or crinkle chips, which hold more fat.

* If you are tempted by a side order, share it with someone else so that you are not restricting yourself but are only consuming half the portion.

* If you're ordering Chinese, go for lower-fat dishes like steamed fish, chicken chop suey and Sichuan prawns. Avoid sweet-and-sour pork and anything fried in batter.

* Ask for a side salad and eat it with your main meal to help fill you up.

* Try sushi and healthy wraps instead of shop-bought sandwiches, which are generally high in calories and loaded with high-fat spreads and mayonnaise.

* Swap a whole-milk latte for a small soya or coconut latte. Avoid syrups and flavourings (unless sugar free) as these can add extra sugar.

* Eat slowly and consciously.

Motivation to Exercise

Thank you. I gained a lot of weight following a major lifestyle change last June and have decided that today is the day to start my journey back to my target weight. You have given me the 'push' I need to start this new phase of my journey.

Karen H.

Finding and maintaining the motivation to exercise can be difficult for some. Everyone wants to be in great shape and to look good, but the journey can appear daunting. For many, joining a gym can be a scary prospect, with the thought of unfamiliar machines, unfamiliar people and feeling self-conscious. For others, health issues or affordability can hinder the ability to exercise.

There are, however, things you can do to overcome the barriers that may stand in your way, helping you to become healthier, fitter and lighter. The fact is that a little movement goes a long way, even if you are only able to do this from your chair.

Vision board

Create a vision board. Either find a photograph of yourself when you were at a weight you would like to return to or find a 'realistic' picture of how you would like to look and pin it to your board.

You should also write your weight goal on your vision board and use Post-it notes or a chart to document the reduction in your size in centimetres, inches, pounds or kilograms. Keep your vision board in a visible place, where you can look at it and appreciate it daily. This will help to keep you focused.

Clear goals

Create clear and realistic goals of what you would ultimately like to achieve. This could be a dress size you wish to fit into, the number of centimetres or inches you would like to lose from your waist or thighs or an ideal weight.

Note down small targets on your journey to give you a sense of achievement, and also reward yourself with little treats along the way. You may also want to consider taking part in organised charity walks, runs or bike rides as part of your health journey, as that will benefit a good cause as well as you.

Buddy up

We will often do more for others than we will do for ourselves, which is why exercising with a friend is a great way to keep you both on track and motivated to keep going. Some people also respond better to healthy competition, therefore sharing your journey and competing with each other can give you both a boost.

Book classes/diarise your exercises

If you have a hair or dental appointment, you are likely to write this appointment in your diary or on a wall calendar, so that you see it through and don't forget it. Should someone ask you to do something that clashes with these appointments, you are likely to decline and offer them an alternative.

We would recommend you use the same process with

your exercise routine. Write it in your diary as if it were an appointment, or book yourself a place in an organised class, and then put a lovely big tick at the side of it when you have completed your exercise.

Group exercise

Group exercise usually consists of people of all different ages, shapes and sizes. It is also a great opportunity to meet new friends, and is often more fun and motivating than exercising alone. Local gyms, swimming baths, churches and social clubs will offer a variety of options for a variety of fitness levels. If there isn't a group that suits you, however, perhaps consider starting your own walking, dancing, swimming or cycling group.

At home

The dictionary definition of exercise is 'physical activity that you do to make your body strong and healthy'.[38] There is no mention of gyms or aerobic classes, just physical activity, and that can take whatever form you wish. It could mean hoovering, gardening, walking up and down your stairs – even choreographing your own dance routine to your favourite music in the comfort and privacy of your own home, or from a chair if you struggle with mobility.

You can also use everyday household items to help build strength, such as food cans, water bottles or even your baby (being very careful). Eva would hold our children when they were babies while doing squats, chest presses and sit-ups, and would also power-walk while taking them for a walk in their pushchairs.

Weight-lifting is a significant component to weight loss, health and strength, and should not be underestimated.

Using weights promotes weight loss because muscle helps you burn more calories. The more muscle you have, the higher your metabolic rate.

> **Research shows that your body continues to burn calories after a lifting workout: the lean muscle mass you build from weight-lifting will speed up your resting metabolism . . . You're more likely to burn body fat, instead of muscle, when you lift weights.**
>
> livestrong.com[39]

Finally, if you are one of those people who has an exercise bike hidden under a pile of clothes in your bedroom or sitting in your shed, then how about dusting it down, creating a banging soundtrack and taking two bottles of water for some bicep curls and shoulder presses while cycling? Moving more could be the key to unlocking your permanent health and fitness.

If I'm totally honest, before I attended I thought that I was broken (and, more importantly, unfixable). Now I truly believe that I can grow and learn and make the changes that before I didn't even dare hope for.

Kirsty

13

Your Weight and Your Future

[I] feel a weight lifted just hearing what you had to say and explaining why we get to this point. It just made sense. Lovely people inside and out. xx

Claire W.

Your body is a vehicle that transports you through your life each and every day. You would never intentionally put diesel in a petrol car, or vice versa, as it would damage your car and severely affect how it runs. You ensure your car has water and oil, that it is serviced annually and that everything is in good working order to keep you safe, especially if you are going to take it on a long journey. You should treat your body in the same way – after all, it is the only vehicle you will ever have, it is with you for your longest journey ever – one that will last your entire lifetime – and therefore it is your responsibility to respect it and make sure it is running well by putting in only the best possible fuel.

We would encourage you to remember this analogy every time you are about to add fuel to your body. Respect, love and be grateful for your body, this amazing vehicle that holds you together, supports you and carries you through life, allowing you to create so many beautiful and amazing memories. When you really appreciate your body and realise how wonderfully remarkable you are, caring for it can become effortless.

Saboteurs

People

There may be people in your life who will sabotage your weight-loss success, so be aware of them among those you live, work and socialise with. You may hear them make statements such as 'one won't do you any harm', 'don't be boring', 'you're losing too much weight' or 'you've changed', among other comments, to try to encourage you to eat something that you know will derail your new healthy-eating plan.

People who are unsupportive are generally so because:

* **they are envious of your positive changes and weight-loss success.**

* **they have issues with food themselves and want you to join them so as to justify their own overeating.**

* **they fear they may lose you, because as you and they will notice, when your weight decreases your confidence increases.**

* **they have low self-esteem, and you looking and feeling better makes them feel worse about themselves.**

Should anyone be unsupportive or try to sabotage your weight-loss success, appreciate that this is a compliment, for they have realised that you are succeeding, you've taken control and you are looking great. When it's clear someone has taken control of their life, it does often make people around them feel inadequate, as they worry they would not be able to do the same.

Again, never forget that only you will be with you every moment of every day for the rest of your life, and your health and happiness is all that matters. When you are happy, healthy, confident and strong then you can do more for yourself, your loved ones and others. Life is amazing, and to enjoy it as much as possible we should strive not only for longevity, but to be fit, healthy and mobile during that time.

Excuses

Perhaps the greatest saboteurs you will face will be the excuses you may use to justify to yourself eating unhealthy foods and not exercising.

Common excuses are:

* **I have no willpower.**
* **I can start again on Monday.**
* **I can start again tomorrow.**
* **One won't hurt.**
* **I'm too busy.**
* **I'm tired.**

Acknowledging that these statements are excuses is the first step. The second is understanding why you may be looking for an excuse to sabotage your weight loss in the first place. The third is appreciating that you are not dieting or restricting yourself, therefore a little of something unhealthy occasionally is okay – once a week perhaps – particularly if you're drinking lots of water and exercising.

However, if you feel you do not have enough willpower, understand that desire creates willpower, so make sure you have followed our motivational tips in Chapter 12 of creating a vision board, having clear, defined goals, changing negative schemas from your past and boosting your self-esteem.

If not having the time is an issue, try to find somewhere close to your office where you could exercise during your lunch hour or before starting work. Also, remember that exercise does not have to take place in a gym, so why not make those calls while taking a brisk walk? The value of time is equal to all, so if one person can make time, then you can too, even if you have to address your time-management skills or learn to delegate and say 'no' occasionally in order to do so.

Finally, if tiredness is the problem, remember that this is a symptom, so ask yourself why you might be tired. There will always be unforeseen events that on occasion take you by surprise and result in a poor or broken night's sleep. But if you are frequently tired, consider why and how this can be rectified. You may need to visit your GP for blood tests. When you begin to drink more water and eat better, your tiredness should improve. Exercise should give you more energy, and having 15-minute power naps could help, too.

Hydration

Drinking water helps boost your metabolism, flushes waste from your body and acts as an appetite suppressant. Drinking plenty of water also encourages your body to stop retaining water, which helps you to lose the additional water weight you are likely to be carrying if you do not drink enough.

The hypothalamus is the part of your brain that regulates your appetite and thirst, and when you are dehydrated, the messaging signals in the hypothalamus become crossed, leading to you feeling hungry when all you actually need is a drink of water. It is therefore essential to your weight-loss success that you are always adequately hydrated (see Chapter 5, page 80).

When we first started to train ourselves to drink more water, we began by drinking a pint of water in the morning, and we would then not allow ourselves to drink our usual daytime drinks of tea or coffee unless we drank a pint of water first. Once you start drinking more water, you will notice that at first you are running back and forth to the toilet, but this is a brilliant leap forward, as you are losing waste, reducing water retention and burning extra calories as you run to the toilet!

You will soon develop a new habit and find that you want to drink water without having to make a conscious effort. We now carry a bottle of water everywhere we go and pack a 2-litre bottle in each of our suitcases if we're travelling to ensure we have our quota for our first night away.

Though it depends on age, humans are on average made of approximately 60 per cent water. Blood is 90 per cent water, your brain and heart are made of 73 per cent water, lungs 83 per cent and muscles and kidneys 79 per cent.[40] So as well as keeping your appetite in check and aiding additional effortless weight loss, drinking water is essential to maintaining healthy skin, organs and bodily functions.

CASE STUDY
John: Weight Loss with Water

John attended one of our workshops and returned nine months later, having lost a significant amount of weight. After congratulating him on the fact that he looked so well, we enquired as to how he had made such a difference in a relatively short space of time.

John explained that he came from a large Spanish family and that eating food was a significant part of his family life – they would get together at his grandmother's home every weekend, and had done ever since he was a little boy. He added that, although he was never slim, he had slowly gained weight over the years as his lifestyle had started to slow down. Now that he was married and working in an office where he was sat at a desk all day, his movement had significantly reduced. After attending our workshop, however, he recalled that we suggested people should be more hydrated, as most do not drink enough water. He said he was most definitely guilty of this, as he rarely drank water and drank a lot of coffee instead. Coffee is a diuretic, which means that it stimulates the increased formation of urine, thereby contributing to subsequent dehydration.

As we had suggested, after starting to drink more water, John would not allow himself to drink coffee unless he drank a large glass of water first. As a result, he slowly found himself drinking more water than coffee as he trained himself to create this new habit.

He told us that at first this change had made him need the toilet a lot, but now this had regulated. The most significant difference he had noticed, however, was that simply by drinking more water – and doing nothing else – he had lost weight. This development had then led him to be more active, because he had more energy. The month before, he had even joined a gym.

We were delighted to hear that just one small, simple change had had such a significant impact on John. We are confident that now he has started to attend a gym as well, the next time we see him he will be looking even healthier, slimmer and fitter.

The Foods You Eat

I attended the London workshop and had to let you know that after seeing the section on dairy, I haven't touched milk or cheese. I not only stopped eating dairy, I've also gone off chocolate. What a fantastic turn I've taken, thanks to you guys. I had the best day ever. Love you all for making it possible. x

Tina M.

No restrictive diet is effective long term, and one of the main reasons for this is that they are often based on foods you would not normally eat. Your food diary will give you a good indication of the foods and dishes you enjoy and eat often. You will also recall that we encouraged you to start writing a shopping list in Chapter 5 (see page 79), based on finding healthier substitutions for the things you love. It is a good idea to have a basic, go-to shopping list to ensure you always have a supply of healthier options in the house, because what you have in your cupboards is what you will eat. And if you order your groceries online, all the better, as this will help diminish the temptations.

Shopping

Here are some tips to help you construct your permanent healthy shopping list, using some healthier alternatives:

* **Make a shopping list and stick to it, or better still, shop online.**

* Choose dairy-, fat- and sugar-free items for your list.

* Soya or coconut milk yoghurts and desserts are a good alternative to dairy.

* Try sugar-free jelly, made with ½ pint of sugar-free lemonade for a fizzy, more interesting taste, or make trifle using low-fat soya custard and a dollop of coconut vanilla yoghurt on top.

* Add kitchen roll to your shopping list, as it's a great fat-soaking tool.

* Use soya spreads or avocado instead of butter.

* If you like savoury snacks, try plain or flavoured rice cakes or gluten-free crackers. Spread crackers with avocado or low-fat hummus.

* If you like chips now and then, go for thick-cut chips or thick-cut carrots lightly sprayed with oil, sprinkled with a little salt and roasted in the oven.

Shopping list

Here's an example of our shopping list:

Reusable water bottle

Fruit – apples, oranges, pears, plums, blueberries, strawberries, melon

Salad – lettuce, tomatoes, cucumber, celery, radish

Vegetables – onions, garlic, carrots, broccoli, spinach, asparagus, kale, parsnips, mushrooms, butternut squash, courgette

Avocado (use this as a replacement for butter)

Sweet potatoes and yams

Natural raw almonds

Small boxes of raisins

Cold-pressed extra-virgin olive oil

Low-calorie cooking oil (spray)

Balsamic vinegar

Gluten-free or pumpernickel bread

Gluten-free wraps

Organic peanut butter/ almond or cashew nut butter

Brown rice

Gluten-free pasta

Rice cakes

Soya yoghurts or coconut milk yoghurt

Unsweetened almond, oat, coconut or soya milk

Low-fat soups

Tinned beans

Tomato-based pasta sauces

Tinned tomatoes

Gluten-free crackers

Free-range eggs

Oats

Cinnamon

Quorn/Quorn products

Frozen spinach, broccoli and frozen vegetables to make soup

Chicken and turkey breast

Chicken and turkey mince

Cooked or sliced chicken and turkey

Oily fish e.g. mackerel

Fresh and tinned fish

Dried and fresh herbs, black pepper

Kitchen roll, to absorb excess oil

Nik and Eva made my 2017 . . . Since meeting them I've lost a stone in weight.

Katie

14

Recipes

I'll be forever grateful for having the opportunity to come and see you yesterday. Thanks so much for everything . . . you had the answers before I even had the question.

Katie E.

In 1998, when we made the decision to be healthy and subsequently opened our health club, we wanted our members to eat healthily like we did. So, as a 'foodie' and someone who adores cooking, Eva created some recipes based on healthier alternatives for the foods we enjoyed.

Of course, we are not nutritionists, and you should always seek medical advice before embarking on any new eating plan. This chapter is simply based upon what worked for us and our health-club members.

Breakfast Options

* 60g/2oz porridge oats made with hot water or soya, coconut or almond milk, a drizzle of honey and a sprinkle of cinnamon and optional fruit (raspberries or blueberries)

* 2 Quorn sausages with spinach

* 1 slice of gluten-free or rye-bread toast with 3 poached or scrambled egg whites or 1 mushroom omelette (made with egg whites only)

* 1 slice of gluten-free or rye-bread toast with 3 slices of turkey

* 3 slices of turkey bacon, 1 poached egg and 2 tablespoons of low-sugar baked beans

* 1 orange, apple or pear with 2 slices of sugar-free, fat-free fruit cake (see page 278) or malt loaf

* 1 banana, 1 tangerine and 1 small bag of dried fruit and nuts (not sugared or salted)

* 2 crisp breads with avocado or peanut butter, with raisins and 1 apple or pear

* Healthy Sunday fry-up! 3 slices of grilled turkey bacon, 1 grilled tomato, 5 grilled mushrooms, 2 tablespoons of low-sugar baked beans and 1 egg-white omelette

Lunch Options

All lunch options can include unlimited vegetables, such as broccoli, spinach, carrots or green beans, or salad, undressed or with a light dressing.

* 1 baked potato with 1 tin of tuna or mackerel, followed by 1 orange or tangerine or 1 handful of grapes

* 1 chicken breast or fish steak (uncoated, so no batter or breadcrumbs) with 1 small sweet potato, followed by 1 tangerine or orange

* 1/2 cereal bowl of brown rice or 3/4 cereal bowl of gluten-free pasta with a tomato sauce (no cheese), followed by 1/2 melon

* 1 baked potato or sweet potato with 1/2 tin of low-sugar baked beans

* Homemade soup with 2 slices of gluten-free bread, 2 crisp breads or 60g/2oz brown rice (optional), followed by 1 small banana or 1 handful of grapes

* 1 gluten-free tortilla wrap with sliced turkey, chicken breast, tuna or mackerel and salad, followed by 1 tangerine or 1 handful of strawberries

* 3 slices of turkey bacon, 1 poached egg, 2 tablespoons of low-sugar baked beans and 1 slice of gluten-free toast (optional), followed by 1 orange

* Mushroom and spinach omelette (made with 3 eggs whites) and 1 slice of gluten-free toast (optional) spread with avocado, followed by 1 apple

* Large bowl of salad with chopped tomatoes, 1/2 avocado, turkey, chicken or turkey ham, 1 boiled egg and a light dressing or homemade vinaigrette, followed by 1 apple or pear

Dinner Options

Choose one starter and one main meal, or one main meal and one dessert.

STARTER (choose one)

* 5 chicken breast tikka bites

* 1/2 melon

* Clear or vegetable soup

* Prawns and salad with lemon juice or very light homemade prawn-cocktail sauce (2 teaspoons of low-fat mayonnaise with a drop of ketchup)

* Egg-white omelette with salad (using 2 eggs)

MAIN COURSE (choose one)

All options can be served with unlimited steamed broccoli, spinach, carrots, asparagus or salad, either undressed or with a light dressing.

Omit simple carbohydrates after 7 p.m. (no rice or potatoes). Add extra vegetables, roasted butternut squash or carrot, or courgette, onion and mushroom mix, lightly sprayed with oil and a little salt and pepper.

You can choose any of the lunch options, or from the dinner options below:

* Grilled chicken, turkey or fish with 1 large or 2 small baked or boiled sweet potatoes or 60g/2oz brown rice and vegetables

* Chicken stir-fry with lots of veggies and rice noodles

* Lean grilled lamb with no fat (no more than once a week) with 1 large or 2 small sweet potatoes or 60g/2oz brown rice

* Gluten-free pasta with a tomato-based sauce (cereal-bowl size)

* 60g/2oz brown rice with stir-fried vegetables and chicken

* Braised turkey or chicken in a sauce, such as a low-calorie soup or tinned tomatoes with stock cubes. Put in a slow-cooker with fresh herbs, onions and mushrooms in the morning

* Homemade **meatloaf** or **meatballs** made with turkey or chicken mince (see recipe on page 262)

* **Spaghetti bolognaise** made with turkey or chicken mince (see page 256)

* Chilli made with turkey or chicken mince and low-sugar baked beans

DESSERT
(choose one to accompany a main meal)

Omit all carbohydrates after 7 p.m.

* 1 small pot of soya or coconut yoghurt

* 25g/1oz oats mixed with natural soya yoghurt, 1 small box of raisins and some blueberries, sprinkled with cinnamon

* 1 slice of fat-free, sugar-free fruit cake (see page 278) or honey loaf (see page 279)

* Natural nuts and raisins (1 large handful)

* 2 large caramel rice cakes

* 5 **Almond balls** (see page 268)

* Fat-free jelly with low-fat custard (preferably soya or dairy-free) and fruit in natural juice

* Sugar-free Angel Delight made with almond or soya milk

* 1/2 melon with strawberries, sprinkled with cinnamon

* 1 handful of grapes, 1 tangerine and 1 orange

SNACKS

For a mid-morning or afternoon snack (optional).

* 1 small bag of dried fruit (prunes, apricots, etc.)

* 1 small banana (no more than 1 a day) or 1 apple or pear

* 1 small pot of soya or coconut yoghurt

* 1 plain chicken breast

* 2 crisp breads with a thin layer of peanut butter, honey or avocado

* 1 tin of mackerel with 2 crisp breads

* 1 boiled egg and 2 crisp breads or 2 slices of gluten-free toast with avocado

* Punnet of strawberries

* 2 rice cakes

DRINKS

DRINK LOTS OF WATER.

* Herbal teas (green, nettle, peppermint and dandelion teas are excellent)

* Iced sparkling water with lemon

* Water infused with fresh lemon, fresh mint and cucumber, raspberries, strawberries or sliced orange

Eva's Recipes

LENTIL (OR TURKEY) BOLOGNAISE

SERVES 6

INGREDIENTS

Drop of olive oil or 2–3 squirts of low-calorie cooking spray

1 onion, chopped

2 garlic cloves, crushed

2 carrots, grated

2 sticks of celery, chopped

500g/17.5oz cooked green lentils/1 pack of lean turkey mince

400g/14oz tin of chopped tomatoes

2 tablespoons tomato purée

400ml/³/₄ pint of vegetable stock

1 tablespoon fresh marjoram or 1 teaspoon dried

1 teaspoon oregano

Black pepper, to taste

METHOD

1 Heat the oil in a non-stick pan, then wipe away the excess with kitchen roll.

2 Quick-fry the onion for 2 minutes, then add the garlic, carrots and celery and fry for a further 5 minutes, adding a splash of water if they are sticking to the pan.

3 Add the lentils (or turkey mince, if using), chopped tomatoes, tomato purée, stock, herbs and pepper, then bring the mix to the boil. Partially cover the pan and simmer for 20–25 minutes (longer if using turkey mince) until thickened.

4 Serve with gluten-free pasta, brown rice or a jacket
   potato.

ALOO GOBI

SERVES 4

INGREDIENTS

450g/1lb sweet potatoes or yams cut in 2.5cm/1in chunks

Drop of olive oil or 2–3 squirts of low-calorie cooking spray

1 teaspoon cumin seeds

1 green chilli, deseeded and finely chopped

450g/1lb cauliflower, broken into florets

1 teaspoon ground coriander

1 teaspoon cumin

¼ teaspoon chilli powder

½ teaspoon turmeric

½ vegetable stock cube

Fresh coriander, to garnish (optional)

METHOD

1 Parboil the potatoes for approximately 10 minutes, drain,
   then set aside.

2 Heat the oil in a non-stick pan, then wipe away the excess
   with kitchen roll. Fry the cumin seeds for 2 minutes, then
   add the green chilli and fry for a further 1 minute.

3 Add the cauliflower florets and fry for a further 5 minutes.

4 Add the potatoes and the spices, then sprinkle over the
   stock cube and continue to fry for a further 7–10 minutes.

5 Garnish with the coriander (if using) and serve either
   alone or with pitta bread or rice and vegetables.

LENTIL BIRYANI

SERVES 4

INGREDIENTS

140g/5oz red lentils

115g/4oz brown basmati rice

Drop of olive oil or 2–3 squirts of low-calorie cooking spray

4 cloves

¼ teaspoon cumin seeds

1 large onion, thinly sliced

1 large sweet potato, cut into 2.5cm/1in chunks

¼ teaspoon turmeric

½ vegetable stock cube

300ml/½ pint of water

METHOD

1 Wash the lentils and rice in several changes of cold water, then leave in a bowl of water to soak for 15 minutes.

2 Heat the oil in a non-stick pan and wipe away the excess with kitchen roll, then add the cloves and cumin seeds and fry for approximately 2 minutes until the seeds start to splutter.

3 Add the onion and potato and fry for a further 5 minutes.

4 Drain the lentils and rice and add to the pan, followed by the turmeric, then sprinkle over the stock cube and fry for a further 5 minutes.

5 Add the water, then bring to the boil and simmer gently for about 20 minutes until the water has been absorbed and the potatoes are tender.

6 Leave to stand, covered, for a further 10 minutes before serving.

KIDNEY BEAN CURRY

SERVES 4

INGREDIENTS

225g/8oz dried kidney beans (or cheat with 2 small tins)

Drop of olive oil or 2–3 squirts of low-calorie cooking spray

$1/2$ teaspoon cumin seeds

1 onion, thinly sliced

1 green chilli, deseeded and finely chopped

2 garlic cloves, crushed

2.5cm/1in piece of fresh root ginger, grated

2 tablespoons curry powder or low-fat curry paste

1 teaspoon cumin

1 teaspoon ground coriander

$1/2$ teaspoon chilli powder

$1/2$ vegetable stock cube

400g/14oz tin of chopped tomatoes

2 tablespoons fresh coriander, to garnish (optional)

METHOD

1 Soak and cook the dried kidney beans as per the instructions or rinse and drain the tinned variety thoroughly.

2 Heat the oil in a non-stick pan and wipe away the excess with kitchen roll, then add the cumin seeds and fry for 2 minutes. Add the onion, chilli, garlic and ginger and fry for a further 5 minutes.

3 Stir in the curry powder or paste, the cumin, ground coriander, chilli powder and stock cube and cook for a further 5 minutes.

4 Add the chopped tomatoes and then simmer for 5 minutes.

5 Add the kidney beans and half of the fresh coriander (if using), adding water if needed.

6 Serve with rice and sprinkle with the remaining fresh coriander (if using) and a tablespoon of low-fat natural yoghurt if desired.

TURKEY PASTA BAKE

SERVES 4

INGREDIENTS

280g/10oz lean turkey mince

1 pack of smoked turkey bacon rashers, chopped

2 garlic cloves, crushed

1 onion, finely chopped

2 carrots, diced

2 tablespoons tomato purée

Handful of fresh basil

300ml/½ pint of chicken stock

225g/8oz gluten-free pasta

Black pepper, to taste

METHOD

1 Brown the mince in a non-stick pan, with a little spray oil or water, then add the turkey bacon, garlic, onion, carrots, tomato purée, basil and black pepper to taste.

2 Add the stock, then bring to the boil, cover and simmer for 1 hour.

3 Preheat oven to 180°C/350°F/Gas 4.

4 Cook the pasta in salted water until al dente. Drain thoroughly, then mix with the turkey mixture.

5 Transfer to a shallow ovenproof dish and bake for 20–30 minutes.

TURKEY AND TOMATO HOTPOT

SERVES 4

INGREDIENTS

30g/1oz gluten-free bread

2 tablespoons soya milk

1 garlic clove, crushed

$^1/_2$ teaspoon caraway seeds

225–280g/8–10oz lean turkey mince

1 egg white

350ml/12fl oz of chicken stock

400g/14oz tin of chopped tomatoes

1 tablespoon tomato purée

115g/4oz brown rice (easy cook)

Fresh basil

Black pepper and sea salt, to taste

METHOD

1 Cut the bread into tiny cubes and put in a mixing bowl with the soya milk and soak for 5 minutes.

2 Add the garlic, caraway seeds and turkey mince to the bowl, then add lots of pepper and the slightest amount of sea salt.

3 In a separate bowl, whisk the egg white until stiff and then fold into the turkey mixture. Leave to chill for 10 minutes.

4 Put the stock, chopped tomatoes and purée into a large pan and bring to the boil.

5   Thoroughly rinse the rice several times, then add to the tomato mixture. Boil for 5 minutes, then reduce to a simmer.

6   Now shape the chilled turkey mixture into approximately 16 balls and drop them into the tomato sauce. Simmer for 15–20 minutes until the turkey and rice are cooked.

7   Garnish with basil and serve with a warm granary baguette.

MEATLOAF
(or use the same mix to make meatballs)

SERVES 4

INGREDIENTS

1 pack of turkey bacon (to line tin)

280g/10oz lean turkey mince

100g/4oz cooked brown rice, rinsed (optional)

6 egg whites, lightly whisked, or liquid egg white

1 large onion, chopped

1 garlic clove, crushed

$1/2$ teaspoon paprika

1 tablespoon mustard

1 tablespoon ketchup

1 vegetable stock cube

400g/14oz tin of chopped tomatoes

Handful of fresh basil

Black pepper, to taste

METHOD

1   Grease a 1.5l/2lb loaf tin and line with baking parchment. Preheat the oven to 180°C/350°F/Gas 4.

2   Cut the turkey bacon rashers into 3 long strips and line the tin with them, saving some for the topping.

3   Blend the remaining ingredients together in a bowl with your hands and then place the mixture into the loaf tin.

4   Cover with the remaining turkey bacon and a piece of baking parchment.

5   Bake in the oven for 1½ hours.

LOW-FAT HUMMUS

INGREDIENTS

400g/14oz tin of chickpeas, rinsed and drained

1 garlic clove

Juice of 1 lemon

1 avocado, stoned, peeled and cut into chunks

½ teaspoon paprika

2 tablespoons extra-virgin olive oil (optional)

Black pepper, to taste

METHOD

Place all ingredients in a blender and blitz to make a smooth paste. You may need to add a little water for a smooth consistency.

GUACAMOLE

INGREDIENTS

3 or 4 avocados, stoned, peeled and chopped into chunks

Juice of 1 lemon

2 garlic cloves, crushed

1 tablespoon cold-pressed, extra-virgin olive oil (optional)

Dash of Tabasco sauce (optional)

Dash of soy sauce (optional)

1 onion, chopped

1 jalapeño pepper, deseeded and chopped

2 large tomatoes, diced

1 teaspoon chilli powder

1 teaspoon paprika

METHOD

1 Blend or mash the avocado with the lemon juice, garlic, olive oil, Tabasco and soy sauce (if using).

2 Mix in the remaining ingredients for a coarse guacamole.

3 If you prefer a smooth guacamole, blend all the ingredients (except for the tomatoes, chilli and paprika, which you can sprinkle over the guacamole at the end).

4 Use as a dip for crudités or lightly toasted rye bread.

PASTA WITH TURKEY MEATBALLS

SERVES 4

INGREDIENTS

450g/1lb lean turkey mince

85g/3oz gluten-free breadcrumbs (make your own using dried gluten-free bread)

1 tablespoon chopped fresh parsley

1 onion, very finely chopped

$1/2$ teaspoon dried thyme

1 teaspoon mustard or ketchup

1 tablespoon cold-pressed, extra-virgin olive oil

1 tablespoon plain gluten-free flour

300ml/ $1/2$ pint of chicken stock

400g/14oz tin of chopped tomatoes

Dash of Worcestershire sauce

2 garlic cloves, crushed

Black pepper, to taste

METHOD

1   Mix together the turkey mince, breadcrumbs, parsley, onion, thyme, mustard (or ketchup), half of the crushed garlic and a pinch of black pepper, then shape the mixture into approximately 24 small balls.

2   Heat the olive oil in a non-stick pan, then wipe away the excess with kitchen roll. Stir in the flour and heat for about 1 minute.

3   Stir in the stock, then add the chopped tomatoes, the rest of the crushed garlic and the remaining ingredients. Stir over the heat until sauce thickens and comes to the boil slightly.

4 Reduce the heat and then simmer, adding the meatballs. Spoon the sauce over the meatballs and allow to simmer for 30 minutes or until the meat is cooked.

5 Meanwhile, cook the pasta of your choice in salted water as per the instructions, then drain and serve with the meatballs and sauce.

TOMATO AND CHICKPEA SOUP

SERVES 4

INGREDIENTS

1 onion, finely chopped

1 stick of celery, finely chopped

1/2 red pepper, deseeded and chopped

1/2 tablespoon cold-pressed, extra-virgin olive oil

1 tablespoon tomato purée

1 tablespoon sugar replacement such as Stevia/
   2 tablespoons pineapple juice (optional)

400g/14oz tin of chopped tomatoes

100g/3 1/2oz red lentils, rinsed

500ml/17fl oz of low-salt chicken stock

400g/14oz tin of chickpeas, rinsed and drained

Juice of 1/2 lemon

Handful of fresh coriander, roughly chopped

METHOD

1 In a food processor, blitz the onion, celery and red pepper to a purée, then heat the oil in a non-stick pan, wiping away the excess with kitchen roll, and cook the purée for 5 minutes.

2 Stir in the tomato purée and sugar replacement or juice (if using).

3 Add the chopped tomatoes and lentils to the pan, along with the stock.

4 Bring to the boil, then cover and simmer for 30 minutes.

5 After 30 minutes, add the chickpeas and cook for a further 5 minutes. Top up with water if necessary.

6 Season to taste and stir through the lemon juice and chopped coriander just before serving.

PARSNIP, SWEET POTATO AND LEEK SOUP

SERVES 4

INGREDIENTS

Drop of olive oil or 2–3 squirts of low-calorie cooking spray
250g/9oz roughly chopped leeks
250g/9oz roughly chopped parsnips
1 sweet potato or small yam, roughly chopped
500ml/17fl oz of low-salt chicken stock
Sprig of fresh thyme

METHOD

1 Heat the oil in a non-stick pan and wipe away the excess with kitchen roll, then add the chopped leeks and cook for 2–3 minutes until soft.

2 Add the parsnips and the potato or yam, stir and then add the stock.

3 Simmer for approximately 25 minutes until the parsnips and potato/yam are cooked, then blitz with a handheld blender.

4 Serve with a sprig of thyme.

SWEET-TREAT ALMOND BALLS

MAKES APPROX. 10–12

INGREDIENTS

100g/3^1/$_2$oz ground almonds

^{1}/$_2$ teaspoon wheatgrass powder (optional, available from health food stores)

^{1}/$_2$ teaspoon cinnamon (optional)

A little honey to bind

METHOD

1 Put the ground almonds in a bowl.

2 Add the wheatgrass and cinnamon (if using).

3 Add the honey a little at a time. Knead the mixture (adding more honey as needed) until it sticks together like dough.

4 Break off small pieces of the dough and roll between your hands to form small bite-sized balls that are then ready to eat.

SLOW-COOKER CHICKEN AND MUSHROOM CURRY

SERVES 4

INGREDIENTS

4 skinless chicken breasts, chopped into chunks

Few drops of soy sauce, for frying

1 onion, finely chopped

294g/10oz tin of low-fat, condensed mushroom soup

150g/5^1/$_2$oz mushrooms, sliced

2 teaspoons curry powder

2 teaspoons mixed dried herbs

1 vegetable stock cube (optional)

METHOD

1 Place the chicken in a non-stick frying pan and fry in a little water and soy sauce until brown on all sides, then transfer to a slow-cooker.

2 Fry the onion as above until softened, then add to the chicken.

3 Place all the remaining ingredients in the slow-cooker and stir. Cook for about 6–8 hours on the low setting.

SLOW-COOKER CHICKEN STEW

SERVES 4

INGREDIENTS

2kg/4 1/2lb lean chicken pieces

3 large carrots, chopped

2 onions, finely chopped

1 garlic clove

400g/14oz tin of chopped tomatoes

2 tablespoons tomato concentrate paste

3 cloves

4 fresh bay leaves

2 tablespoons Worcestershire sauce

1 tablespoon soy sauce

2 tablespoons honey or agave nectar

1 chicken stock cube

500ml/17fl oz water

3 sweet potatoes, peeled and chopped into 2.5cm/1in chunks

METHOD

1 Add the chicken, carrots, onions and garlic to the slow-cooker.

2 Next, add the chopped tomatoes, tomato paste, cloves, bay leaves, Worcestershire and soy sauces, honey, stock cube and water. Stir the ingredients in the slow-cooker to combine.

3 Cover and cook on a low heat for 3 hours, then add the potatoes and top up with more water if necessary.

4 Cook for another 5 or 6 hours.

HEALTHY PROTEIN NUT COOKIES

MAKES 8–10 COOKIES

This is a recipe we throw together at home, using a cup measure to make it easy. We have included the gram and ounce equivalent below.

INGREDIENTS

1 cup (150g/6oz) ground almonds

4–5 tablespoons organic coconut flour

1/2 cup (75g/3oz) pea protein (available from most health food stores)

Stevia, to taste

3–4 tablespoons nut butter

1 cup (150g/6oz) chopped pecans and walnuts

1 cup (150g/6oz) chopped Medjool dates

1 teaspoon vanilla extract

A splash of almond or coconut milk to bind

METHOD

1 Preheat the oven to 180°C/350°F/Gas 4, and spray a baking tray with sunflower or coconut oil.

2 Mix the ground almonds, coconut flour, pea protein and Stevia in a bowl.

3 Add the nut butter and rub into the mixture until it resembles crumbs.

4 Stir in the chopped nuts and dates.

5 Add the vanilla extract, then add a little of the almond or coconut milk to bring the mixture together to form a dough.

6 Rip off small pieces of dough and roll them into balls between your hands, then flatten them to make approximately 8 to 10 cookies.

7 Place the cookies on the greased tray and bake in the oven for around 10 minutes until golden brown.

8 Remove from the oven, leave to cool on a wire rack, then eat – they are delicious!

SWEET MINCEMEAT CAKE BARS

MAKES 8–16 BARS

INGREDIENTS

250g/9oz self-raising gluten-free flour (or plain gluten-free flour plus 2 teaspoons baking powder)

450g/1lb mincemeat (dried fruit variety)

5 egg whites, beaten

2 tablespoons agave nectar

METHOD

1 Preheat the oven to 180°C/350°F/Gas 4, and lightly grease a shallow rectangular baking tin with spray oil.

2 Sift the flour into a large bowl, then stir in the mincemeat, beaten egg whites and agave nectar to combine.

3 Spoon the mixture into the baking tray, then place in the oven and bake for 25–30 minutes until golden brown.

4 Remove from the oven and allow to cool in the tin, then cut into 8 large or 16 smaller bars.

HEALTHY COCONUT AND BLUEBERRY TARTS

MAKES 6

INGREDIENTS

For the tart cases:

100g/3 1/2 oz raw unsalted almonds

90g/3oz plain oatcakes

90g/3oz dried, pitted dates

1 tablespoon coconut oil

2 teaspoons organic maple syrup

Pinch of sea salt

For the filling:

2 1/2 400ml/14fl oz tins of full-fat coconut milk, chilled

3 tablespoons set honey (substitute for an alternative sweetener if you are vegan)

1/2 teaspoon vanilla extract

Pinch of sea salt

200g/7oz blueberries

METHOD

1 Preheat the oven to 200°C/400°F/Gas 6, and line a 6-hole muffin tray with cling film.

2 To make the tart cases, place the almonds on a roasting tray and roast for 5–6 minutes or until they are a shade darker and aromatic, taking care not to let them burn. Then remove from the oven and leave to cool.

3 Place all the ingredients for the cases, including the roasted almonds, in the bowl of a food processor and blitz until the mixture forms a paste that sticks together when you press it between your fingers.

4 Divide the base mixture between the 6 lined muffin holes, pressing it firmly into the bases and sides. Place the muffin tray in the freezer for 20 minutes until the tart cases have set firm, then remove the tray and carefully lift the overhanging cling film from each hole to release the mini tart cases. Place the tart cases on a plate, cover and chill.

5 To make the filling, remove the tins of coconut milk from the fridge without shaking them. Remove the lids and carefully scoop out the very firm, set coconut cream at the top, leaving coconut water in the tins. Add the coconut cream to the cleaned-out bowl of the food processor together with the honey, vanilla extract and salt, then blitz until completely smooth.

6 Remove the tart cases from the fridge and divide the coconut cream filling equally between them. Add a few fresh blueberries to the top of each mini tart.

7 Serve immediately or keep chilled and covered for up to 3 days.

QUICK BANANA AND OAT PANCAKES

SERVES 4

INGREDIENTS

4 ripe bananas

4 eggs

100g/3 1/2 oz gluten-free oats

Pinch of cinnamon

2 teaspoons coconut oil

4 tablespoons dairy-free coconut or soya yoghurt

METHOD

1   In a small bowl, combine the bananas, eggs, oats and cinnamon and mix well.

2   Heat half the coconut oil in a non-stick frying pan over medium heat, then ladle tablespoonfuls of the mixture into the pan to thinly cover the base. Fry the pancakes for 2–4 minutes on each side or until golden brown and cooked through. If you want to make smaller pancakes you should be able to fry 2 or 3 at a time. Repeat with the remaining mixture, adding more oil to the pan if necessary, to make 4 pancakes per person.

3   Serve with the dairy-free coconut yoghurt.

DAIRY-FREE BANANA BERRY ICE CREAM

SERVES 4

INGREDIENTS

4 ripe bananas, peeled and frozen

150g/5 1/2 oz frozen mixed berries or one of your choice, e.g. raspberries or blueberries

75g/2 1/2 oz dairy-free plain, coconut or soya yoghurt

METHOD

1 Place all the ingredients in a food processor and pulse until smooth.

2 Serve straight away or keep in the freezer for up to 40 minutes (after which it will start to freeze solid).

FRUITY FLAPJACKS

MAKES 18 BARS

INGREDIENTS

200g/7oz dried, pitted dates or apricots

100ml/3 1/2 fl oz boiling water

50g/1 3/4 oz nut butter

1 tablespoon honey

150g/5 1/2 oz gluten-free oats

1 tablespoon coconut oil

METHOD

1 Preheat the oven to 200°C/400°F/Gas 6, and line a baking tray (approximately 33 x 23cm/13 x 9in) with baking parchment.

2 Put the dried dates or apricots, water and nut butter into a food processor and blitz. Add the remaining ingredients and pulse a couple of times so that the oats are still chunky but combined.

3 Spoon the mixture into the baking tray and flatten evenly with the back of the spoon. Then bake in the oven for 15 minutes until firm and golden.

4 Remove from the oven and leave to cool slightly in the tin for 10–15 minutes, then loosen the edges with a knife and cut into 18 bars. Remove from the tin and leave to cool completely on a wire rack.

COCONUT CHOCOLATE BITES

MAKES 10 BALLS

INGREDIENTS

75g/2 1/2 oz dried, pitted dates

50g/1 3/4 oz gluten-free oats

50g/1 3/4 oz ground almonds

1 tablespoon cocoa powder

Zest and juice of 1 orange

110g/4oz desiccated coconut

1 tablespoon boiling water

METHOD

1 Place the dates in a glass bowl, cover with boiling water and set aside for 5–10 minutes until soft.

2 Drain any excess water from the dates and place them in a food processor with the oats, ground almonds, cocoa powder and orange zest and juice. Add 75g/2½oz of the desiccated coconut and the boiling water, then blitz until fully combined.

3 With wet hands, roll the mixture into around 10 balls, approximately the size of a golf ball, and then roll them in the remaining desiccated coconut until evenly coated.

HEALTHY PECAN PIE

INGREDIENTS

For the pie case:

180g/6oz chopped pecans

70g/2 1/2 oz unsweetened shredded coconut

150g/5 1/2 oz pitted Medjool dates

For the filling:

200g/7oz pitted Medjool dates

340ml/12fl oz any soya, coconut or almond milk

3 tablespoons arrowroot starch (you can substitute
   with cornstarch or tapioca starch if preferred)

1 teaspoon vanilla extract

¹/₄ teaspoon sea salt

150g/5 ¹/₂oz pecan halves

METHOD

1 Preheat the oven to 180°C/350°F/Gas 4, and line a
   square baking tray (20 x 20cm/8 x 8in) with baking
   parchment.

2 To make the pie case, combine all the ingredients in
   a blender or food processor and blitz until sticky and
   clumpy.

3 Press the case mixture firmly into the baking tray and
   then set aside.

4 To make the filling, blitz the dates, non-dairy milk,
   arrowroot, vanilla extract and salt in the cleaned-out
   blender until smooth.

5 Add ¾ of the pecan halves and pulse them in.

6 Spread the filling mixture on top of the pie case, then
   sprinkle the remaining pecan halves on top and press
   them in lightly.

7 Bake for 35–40 minutes or until the pecans on top are
   golden brown.

8 Remove from the oven and leave to cool before serving.

FAT-FREE, SUGAR-FREE FRUIT CAKE

INGREDIENTS

350g/12oz dried fruit (raisins, cherries, figs, etc.)

225ml/8fl oz cold tea

300g/12oz self-raising gluten-free flour (or plain gluten-free flour plus 2 teaspoons baking powder)

Sugar replacement (manufacturer's equivalent of 150g/6oz for baking) or 5 tablespoons agave nectar

2 egg whites

1 teaspoon mixed spice

2 teaspoons cinnamon

Zest of 1 orange and 1 lemon (optional)

1 teaspoon vanilla essence (optional)

3 tablespoons ground almonds (optional)

Honey or agave nectar, to drizzle (optional)

METHOD

1 Soak the dried fruit in the cold tea overnight.

2 Preheat the oven to 190°C/375°F/Gas 5. Lightly grease a 1.5l/2lb loaf tin, then line with baking parchment sprayed lightly with oil. Leave enough parchment around the edges to be able to cover the top of the cake as well.

3 Blitz all the ingredients, except the ground almonds and honey, in a blender or food processor until combined, then pour the mixture into the loaf tin.

4 Sprinkle the top of the cake with the ground almonds and drizzle with honey or agave nectar (if using).

5 Cover the top of the cake with the extra baking parchment and bake in the oven for 90 minutes. Uncover the top of the cake for the final 20–30 minutes of baking time.

6 Remove from the oven and allow to cool on a wire rack before serving.

LOW-FAT, LOW-SUGAR RAISIN AND HONEY LOAF

INGREDIENTS

300g/10oz plain gluten-free flour

1 1/2 teaspoons baking powder

1/2 teaspoon bicarbonate of soda

1 teaspoon cinnamon

300ml/10fl oz natural soya yoghurt

2 egg whites

60g/2oz raisins

2 tablespoons honey, plus extra to drizzle (optional)

METHOD

1 Preheat the oven to 200°C/400°F/Gas 6. Lightly grease a 1.5l/2lb loaf tin and then line with baking parchment so as not to get any oil in the cake mixture. Leave enough parchment around the edges to be able to cover the top of the cake as well.

2 Mix the flour, baking powder, bicarbonate of soda and cinnamon in a large bowl.

3 Whisk together the yoghurt and egg whites, then gently fold into the flour mixture with the raisins and honey.

4 Spoon the mixture into the loaf tin, drizzle the top of the cake with a little extra honey if desired, then bake in the oven for 20–30 minutes until golden brown.

5 Remove from the oven and allow to cool in the tin for 20–30 minutes, then turn out and serve.

BANANA CAKE

INGREDIENTS

500g/1lb 3oz very ripe bananas

3 egg whites

Sugar replacement (manufacturer's equivalent of 150g/6oz for baking) or 5 tablespoons agave nectar

2 teaspoons cinnamon, plus an extra teaspoon to sprinkle (optional)

Few drops of vanilla extract (optional)

115g/4oz raisins

225g/8oz self-raising gluten-free flour (or plain gluten-free flour plus 2 teaspoons baking powder)

2–4 tablespoons chopped mixed nuts (optional)

1 tablespoon honey, to drizzle (optional)

METHOD

1 Preheat the oven to 180°C/350°F/Gas 4. Lightly grease a 1.5l/2lb loaf tin and then line with baking parchment sprayed lightly with oil. Leave enough parchment around the edges to be able to cover the top of the cake as well.

2 Mash the bananas in a bowl.

3 Whisk the egg whites a little, and then mix in with the banana.

4 Add the sugar replacement, then stir in cinnamon, vanilla extract (if using) and raisins.

5 Fold in the flour, lifting it high to get lots of air into the mixture, and once well combined, pour into the loaf tin.

6 If desired, sprinkle the top with the chopped nuts and the extra cinnamon, then drizzle with the honey (if using).

7   Cover the cake loosely with the extra baking parchment and bake in the oven for 60–70 minutes, uncovering the cake for the final 10 minutes of baking time.

8   Remove from the oven and leave to cool on a wire rack before serving.

SPICED COOKIES

MAKES APPROX. 10–12

INGREDIENTS

140g/5oz soya flour

170g/6oz coconut flour

1 1/2 teaspoons baking powder

1 teaspoon bicarbonate of soda

1/2 teaspoon ground allspice

1 1/4 teaspoons ground ginger

1 1/2 teaspoons cinnamon

225g/8oz frozen apple concentrate, thawed, or 150g/5 1/2 oz fruit spread combined with 75ml/2 1/2 fl oz water

150g/5 1/2 oz dried apricots

2 egg whites

4 tablespoons flaxseed oil

METHOD

1   Combine all the dry ingredients in a mixing bowl.

2   Place the apple concentrate and dried apricots in a blender and blitz at a high speed until the apricots are chopped.

3   Add the egg whites to the blender and pulse slowly until combined.

4   Next, add the wet mixture and the flaxseed oil to the dry ingredients and mix slowly until well combined, to form a soft dough.

5   Wrap the dough in wax paper or baking parchment and place in the fridge to chill for 2 hours.

6   When ready to bake, preheat the oven to 190°C/375°F/ Gas 5.

7   Wet your hands and shape the dough into 4cm/2in balls. Place them on a non-stick baking tray and flatten them with the back of a fork.

8   Bake for 8–10 minutes until just golden.

9   Remove from the oven and allow to cool on a wire rack before eating.

15

Conclusion

At the beginning of this book, we shared with you the essential components for winning at weight loss: addressing your physical, nutritional and mental health and creating a positive environment.

We have endeavoured to cover these areas, and we now pass the baton on to you, because just reading this book is not enough. You have to now take action and put a plan in place to work through your timeline and questionnaire, and carry out our suggestions.

We have shared lots of tips to help motivate you to eat healthily and improve your physical health, as well as encouraging you to consider any environmental issues that could be affecting your weight-loss success. We have also provided techniques for altering your perspective on specific foods that may be sabotaging your good intentions.

We've highlighted how the people around you, together with external factors, can negatively impact you. With our timeline, questionnaire and the many case studies we have given you, we have suggested the possible causes of your negative relationship with food, and have also offered solutions and techniques to help address these causes.

Please make sure that you now create a plan with absolute clarity. Remember that if your plan is just to lose weight, then as soon as you have lost one pound, you will think, 'Job done.' You will have achieved exactly what you said you would, which is why you will then lose motivation without necessarily knowing why.

Having complete clarity in your goal increases your chances of success immensely. Decide exactly what weight or clothes size you want to be and write it down. Don't ever underestimate the power of thought. If you take a look around you right now, everything in your room started with a thought: the sofa you are sitting on, the tables, the carpet or wooden floor – they all began with a thought that then became a reality. And this same kind of creative thinking is the beginning of winning at weight loss.

> **'There is nothing either good or bad but thinking makes it so.'**
>
> **William Shakespeare**

To become the person you really want to be, you have to create a specific, detailed mental picture of that person. If you continue to hold that mental picture in your mind and see it as often as you can, the day will eventually come when you are that person. You must also see yourself doing all the things you need to do to create this image and enjoy your life as that person. Before we do anything, we see it in our minds first.

If you feel like you are falling off the wagon of weight loss, look at your vision board and the positives in your timeline and questionnaire to change your mindset. At the same time, remember that if this happens, a day does not represent your life, and you can start again tomorrow.

However, if the odd days of falling off the wagon become more frequent, look at what is happening in your life. Look for potential emotional triggers. You cannot fix an issue that you are not aware of. Therefore, the first step to succeeding with your weight-loss goals is to understand what barriers stand in your way.

Go back to your timeline to look through your possible triggers but also your successes, to remind yourself of how capable you are. Remember, falling off the wagon does not represent your journey, but it does give you an opportunity to identify what further actions you need to take to perfect your weight-loss journey.

We have shared with you our approach to winning at weight loss, which, in brief, consists of a five-step formula for you to apply to past issues that are negatively affecting your present:

1   Find the original event (the source that created the schema).

2   Consider how you perceived it then.

3   Challenge it with positive evidence to upgrade and condition your negative schema.

4   See the event for what it was through your eyes today, as opposed to how it felt back then.

5   Celebrate that you are not a victim of your past.
    You are a victor of your future.

We very much hope that from the moment you finish reading this book, you will be able to show gratitude towards your body. If you have been unhappy with your weight then undoubtedly you will have felt negative about your body, but from this moment on, we want you to be grateful to the vehicle that carries and supports you each day. Be grateful that you can breathe, be grateful that you are living, be grateful that you are you.

Use our Mirror Technique (see page 148) and love who you are and how you look. Remember that if you have ever been loved, this is because you are lovable. You have earned love and are an incredible human being.

Focus on being healthy, not dieting, and take your time. Work on changing one behaviour at a time, as this will allow the new behaviour to become a habit. You have an exciting journey ahead of you, so to make that journey simpler and easier you must make the decision to enjoy it. While this sounds simplistic, just remember that if you have ever embarked upon a diet before, you probably felt dread as soon as you made the decision, as you felt you would be losing out. But making the decision to move towards a healthier, longer life, which will give you more time with your family and friends and the ability to create more fantastic memories, will make your journey feel thrilling, easy and real.

Acknowledge and celebrate the progress you make on your journey. Enjoy creating a new hobby of health and adopting a new approach to weight loss, and most of all, enjoy loving and respecting the beautiful and unique person you are.

We hope you have enjoyed reading about our work and our personal journey to successful weight loss. It has been a privilege to share with you what has worked for us and so many of our clients, health-club members and workshop delegates.

Wishing you an abundance of health, happiness and success in your weight-loss journey.

Nik & Eva xx

References

1 https://www.nhs.uk/conditions/obesity/

2 https://www.livescience.com/60936-stress-negative-life-events-obesity.html

3 www.nhs.uk/conditions/eating-disorders/

4 https://www.healthline.com/health/celebrities-with-eating-disorders#1

5 https://familydoctor.org/condition/pica/

6 https://www.verywellmind.com/purging-disorder-4157658

7 https://www.beateatingdisorders.org.uk/media-centre/eating-disorder-statistics

8 Piaget, Jean (1952). In E. Boring et al. (eds.), *A History of Psychology in Autobiography*, vol. IV, pp. 237–256. (Worcester, MA: Clark University Press)

9 https://digital.nhs.uk/data-and-information/publications/statistical/statistics-on-obesity-physical-activity-and-diet/statistics-on-obesity-physical-activity-and-diet-england-2019/part-3-adult-obesity

10 https://www.heartuk.org.uk/about-us/media

11 www.bbc.co.uk/news/health-39457993

12 https://www.bhf.org.uk/what-we-do/news-from-the-bhf/news-archive/2017/april/new-report-assesses-impact-of-physical-inactivity-on-uk-heart-health-and-economy

13 https://www.ihrsa.org/about/media-center/press-releases/
u-s-physical-activity-study-shows-28-of-americans-inactive/

14 www.thensmc.com/resources/showcase/change4life

15 https://researchbriefings.files.parliament.uk/documents/
SN03336/SN03336.pdf

16 https://www.nhs.uk/conditions/obesity/

17 www.independent.co.uk/news/science/archaeology/300000-
year-old-firepit-found-in-israel-could-be-the-first-example-of-
a-social-campfire-9091822.html

18 https://www.eatthis.com/side-effects-of-msg-increased-
appetite-weight-gain-and-more/

19 https://www.healthline.com/nutrition/drinking-water-helps-
with-weight-loss#section4

20 https://www.sciencedaily.com/releases/2018/12/181227111420.
htm

21 https://www.medicalnewstoday.com/articles/320079.php

22 https://www.medicinenet.com/script/main/art.asp?article
key=175310

23 Mitchell, Andie (2015). *It Was Me All Along* (Clarkson Potter).

24 https://www.nbcnews.com/better/business/why-low-self-
esteem-may-be-hurting-your-career-ncna814156

25 https://sites.psu.edu/intropsychs14n1/2014/04/07/taste-
aversion-3/

26 https://www.eurekalert.org/pub_releases/2016-12/uoe-ydm
112916.php

27 http://newsroom.ucla.edu/releases/Dieting-Does-Not-Work-
UCLA-Researchers-7832

28 https://www.ncbi.nlm.nih.gov/pubmed/25614198

29 https://www.eurekalert.org/pub_releases/2016-12/uoe-ydm
112916.php

30 https://eu.usatoday.com/story/news/nation/2012/10/15/sleep-
deprivation-fat-cells/1630289/

31 https://www.bbc.com/news/health-38562048

32 https://www.bbc.com/news/health-38562048

33 https://www.drugabuse.gov/publications/drugs-brains-behavior-science-addiction/drug-misuse-addiction

34 https://www.healthline.com/health/food-nutrition/experts-is-sugar-addictive-drug#1

35 https://www.abbott.co.uk/bin/abbott/SavePageAsPdf.%60content%60abbott%60en-gb%60homepage%60media-center%60news%60children-who-are-fussy-eaters.articlePage.en-gb.pdf

36 http://blog.press.princeton.edu/2017/05/02/alexander-todorov-on-the-science-of-first-impressions/

37 https://www.health.com/health/gallery/0,,20920951,00.html?slide=106005#106005

38 https://dictionary.cambridge.org/dictionary/english/exercise

39 https://www.livestrong.com/article/390546-how-fast-can-you-lose-weight-by-weight-lifting/

40 https://www.healthline.com/health/body-water-percentage#body-water-storage

Charities and Support Groups

http://anxietycare.org.uk

https://www.anxietyuk.org.uk

www.beateatingdisorders.org.uk

https://www.thecalmzone.net

https://www.mind.org.uk

https://www.moodjuice.scot.nhs.uk/posttrauma.asp

www.nhs.uk/conditions/eating-disorders

https://www.nspa.org.uk/members/campaign-living-
    miserably-calm/

https://www.nopanic.org.uk

https://www.oagb.org.uk

https://www.rethink.org

https://www.rcpsych.ac.uk

http://www.samaritans.org

http://www.sane.org.uk

https://youngminds.org.uk

Acknowledgements

Our interest in weight loss, longevity, health and fitness resulted in us opening a health club in 1998. We would like to take this opportunity to thank all of our past members who helped us to identify that weight issues are merely a symptom of a prior thought, which creates a behavioural reference. Thank you to those who shared their life stories with us in order to help us understand and discover the cause of their weight gain.

Those early interactions with our members allowed us to trial our pioneering approach to weight loss, which, due to its success, helped us to write this book – which we sincerely hope will help others.

We would also like to thank our children, Liv and Hunter, who have encouraged and supported us to keep writing, even during our family times. Their understanding of the importance of our work and the need to help others is both heart-warming and hugely appreciated. We are so very proud of them both.

Finally, a huge thank you to Frank Speakman, an incredible man, loving father and the one who ignited us with the love of health and fitness, which has enabled us to help so many.

About the Authors

Nik and Eva Speakman have studied and worked together since 1992, both sharing a passion to help people lead happier and less inhibited lives. Through studying the work of Ivan Pavlov, John Watson, Jean Piaget and B. F. Skinner, they acquired an intellectual curiosity for behaviourism and conditioning. After many breakthroughs, their studies transformed into the creation of their own behavioural change therapy known as 'Schema Conditioning'.

The Speakmans regularly appear on ITV's *This Morning* and have treated clients from all walks of life, including a number of high-profile clients. They are ambassadors and supporters of Variety, the Children's Charity, and they help many people to overcome a wide range of issues through live workshops, tours, books, radio and TV.